CHAIR YOGA
FOR SENIORS OVER
60

Chair Yoga for Weight Loss, Improve Joint Mobility, and Improve Posture | Reclaim Your Youth with Calm Sitting Exercises | 28-Day Challenge Illustration

Ruth Sinclair

COPYRIGHT © 2024 BY RUTH SINCLAIR

The information provided in this book is for educational and informational purposes only. It does not constitute professional advice, and the author and publisher disclaim any liability arising from using this material. Readers should consult relevant professionals for specific advice related to their situations.

TABLE OF CONTENTS

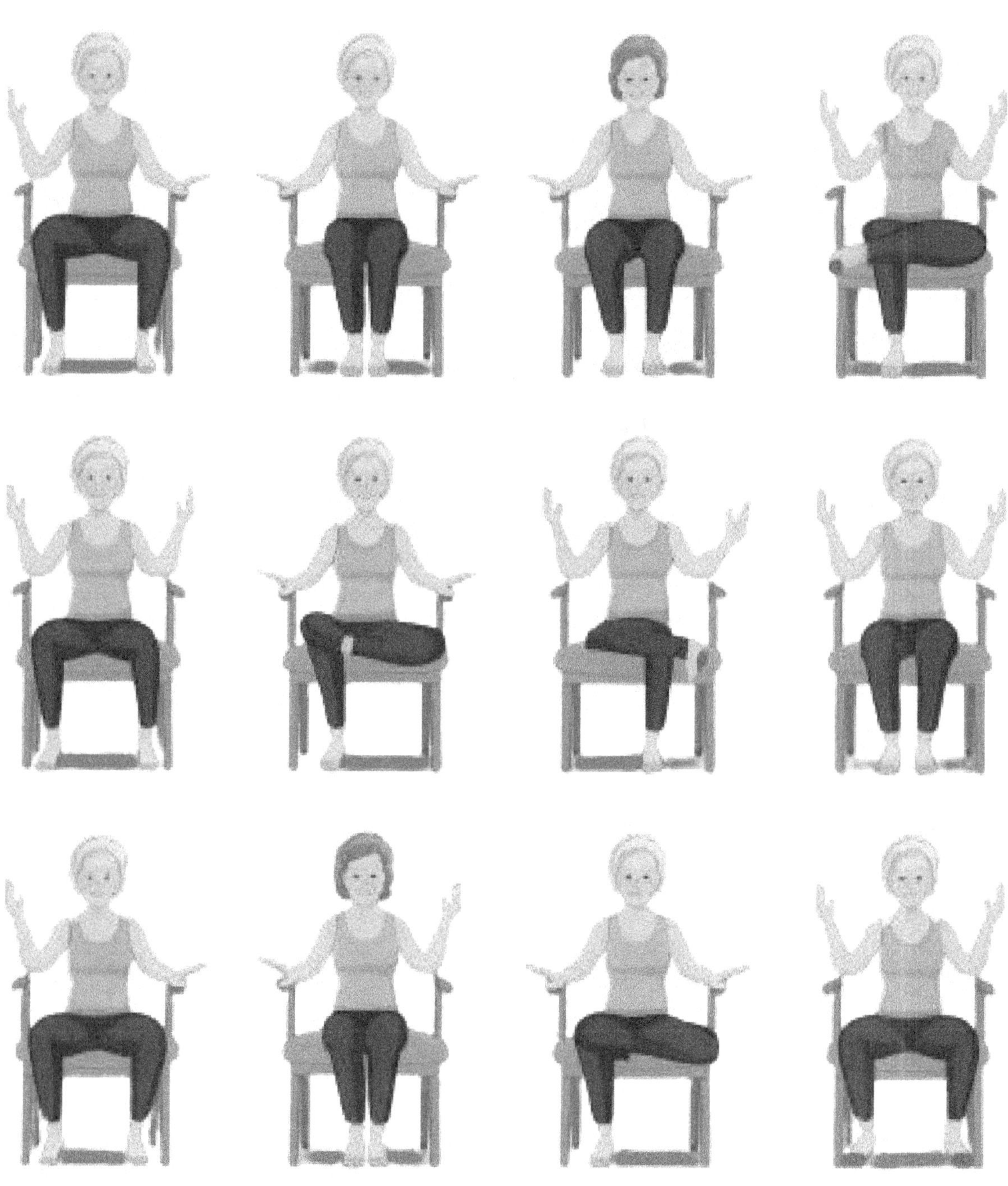

INTRODUCTION

Evelyn's days merged into a repetitive routine of aching joints and muttered moans. At sixty-two her once-vibrant energy had faded, overshadowed by the steady march of time. But then, one rainy afternoon, she bought a book called ***"Chair Yoga for seniors over 60."***

Evelyn traced the engraved letters on the cover, her interest piqued. She sat in her worn armchair, rain pounding on the windowpane, and opened the book. Its pages contained promises of rejuvenation, like murmurs from a distant friend.

The recliner became Evelyn's haven. She followed the directions, raising her arms aloft and feeling the stretch in her back. The book reassured her that even modest gestures were important—that grace could bloom within restrictions.

Evelyn closed her eyes and inhaled deeply. The aroma of paper blended with recollections of the garden she'd nurtured and her late husband's laughter. With each exhale, she released tension, making room for hope.

The chair changed into her companion. Evelyn raised her legs, envisioning roots holding her to the ground. She imagined her granddaughter's face, determined and radiant. "Nana," she'd added, "you're stronger than you know."

As rain fell outside, Evelyn practiced mindfulness. She sipped her morning tea, feeling the warmth on her palms. The book reminded her that being present was a gift she had long ignored.

Evelyn's heart grew. She asked her neighbors to attend her chair yoga sessions. Mrs. Thompson, with her gray hair, giggled as they attempted the tree posture. "We're ancient oaks," she'd add, trembling yet firm.

Evelyn stood up one day instead of sitting in her chair. Her knees trembled, but her soul rose. She danced a slow, methodical waltz around her living room. Raindrops echoed against the roof.

Neighbors peered through the curtains, eyes wide. Evelyn didn't care. She had discovered her rhythm—the music of resilience. The book had become her compass, directing her towards strength, laughter, and connection.

So Evelyn's days changed. She planted flowers in colors that matched the book's images. She wrote letters to old pals, offering details about her unexpected experience. She even taught chair yoga at the community center, and her joy was contagious.

Evelyn sat by the window one evening as the sun began to set. The book was open on her lap, the pages dog-eared and loved. Rainbows swirled across the room, filling the walls with optimism.

Her granddaughter arrived, her eyes wide. "Nana," she remarked, "you're radiant."

Evelyn smiled, her heart like a blossoming lotus. "Grace," she whispered, "is found in the pages we choose to open."

Evelyn's tale evolved, demonstrating tenacity, community, and the transformative power of a simple chair.

CHAPTER 1: INTRODUCTION TO YOGA AND ITS BENEFITS

Yoga is a complete mind-body practice that includes physical postures, breathing exercises, and meditation.

It has become very famous due to its multiple health benefits

Let's look at why yoga is more than simply a workout and how it may improve your well-being.

- ❖ **Physical Health Benefits:**
  - ➢ **Improved Flexibility:** Yoga poses (asanas) stretch and lengthen muscles, resulting in increased flexibility.
  - ➢ **Increased Strength:** Holding postures improves muscle strength, particularly in the core, arms, and legs.
  - ➢ **Better Balance:** Yoga's varied standing and balancing positions help to enhance balance and coordination.
  - ➢ **Increased Bone Density:** Weight-bearing asanas promote bone health and prevent osteoporosis.
  - ➢ **Reduced Chronic discomfort:** Regular practice may help relieve discomfort caused by illnesses such as arthritis.
- ❖ **Mental and Emotional Well-Being:**
  - ➢ **Tension Reduction:** Yoga improves relaxation and decreases tension. It activates parts of the brain associated with joy while decreasing stress-related feelings.
  - ➢ **Improved Mental Focus:** Mindfulness when practicing improves concentration and mental clarity.

- ➢ **Emotional Balance:** Yoga helps with anxiety, depression, and mood swings.
  - ➢ **Energy Boost:** Regular practice raises overall energy levels.
- ❖ **Heart Health and Circulation:**

  blood artery flexibility by up to 69%, potentially lowering arterial blockages.

- ❖ **Other Benefits:**
  - ➢ **Immune System Boost:** Yoga boosts natural antioxidant levels, improving overall immunity.
  - ➢ **Gene Activation:** Even beginners notice favorable improvements in gene expression after 8 weeks of practice.
  - ➢ **Diabetes Management:** Yoga can reduce the requirement for diabetic drugs by up to 40%.
  - ➢ **Fall Prevention:** It promotes equilibrium and may aid in restoring balance after a stumble.
- ❖ **Potential Alzheimer's Prevention:** Meditation in yoga may help to postpone the onset of Alzheimer's and improve memory. Yoga is an effective strategy for promoting overall health.

The mix of physical exercise, breath awareness, and meditation promotes general well-being. People who practice yoga utilize less medical services, lowering their healthcare expenses. So, roll out your mat and experience the transformational power of yoga!

The Origins and History of Yoga

Millions of practitioners worldwide benefit from its physical, mental, and spiritual dimensions.

- ➢ Yoga facilities, retreats, and online platforms provide various practices for people of all ages and backgrounds.

Yoga's evolution from ancient India to the current day exemplifies its versatility, profundity, and transformational force. Whether you're looking for Yoga, a profound practice that combines physical, mental, and spiritual qualities, has a long history spanning over 5,000 years.

Let's look at its fascinating roots.

- ❖ **Ancient Roots:** The Indus-Sarasvati civilization in Northern India is credited with inventing the first forms of yoga.

These rituals began circa 3000 BCE.

- ➢ The term **"yoga"** was originally used in the Rig Veda, the oldest sacred books. These works included hymns, mantras, and rites practiced by Vedic priests (Brahmans).
- ❖ **Pre-Classical Yoga:**
  - ➢ During this time, yoga was mostly an oral practice passed down from teacher to student.
  - ➢ Meditation, breath control, and ethical precepts were the primary focus of the practices.
  - ➢ The Upanishads, philosophical works dating from circa 800 BCE, investigated the nature of reality, awareness, and the self.

They highlighted yoga as a technique of gaining spiritual enlightenment

- ❖ **Classical Yoga:** Patanjali, a sage, composed the 'Yoga Sutras' in the second century CE. These sutras established the foundation of classical yoga.

- ➤ Patanjali's approach defined the eight limbs of yoga (Ashtanga Yoga), which included ethical principles (yamas and niyamas), physical postures (asanas), breath control (pranayama), and meditation (dhyana).
- ➤ Classical yoga sought self-realization, emancipation (moksha), and oneness with the divine.

❖ **Postclassical Yoga**

- ➤ Hatha yoga originated between the ninth and eleventh century CE. It focused on physical postures (asanas) and cleansing practices.
- ➤ Tantric teachings inspired Hatha yoga by introducing energy centers (chakras) and subtle energy conduits (nadis).
- ➤ Hatha yoga literature such as the 'Hatha Yoga Pradipika' and the 'Gheranda Samhita' had thorough directions for asanas, mudras, and pranayama.

❖ **Modern Yoga**

- ➤ In the late 19th and early 20th centuries, Indian masters such as Swami Vivekananda and Paramahansa Yogananda popularized yoga in the Western world.
- ➤ B.K.S. Iyengar, K. Pattabhi Jois, and Indra Devi were influential people who popularized yoga over the world.
- ➤ Modern yoga includes diverse types such as Vinyasa, Bikram, Kundalini, and Iyengar. It focuses on physical health, stress reduction, and relaxation, frequently through asana practice

❖ **Global Impact**

- ➤ Yoga has become a worldwide phenomenon, transcending cultural barriers.

Physical health, mental clarity, or spiritual progress, yoga is a timeless route to wellness.

Understanding Yoga Principles and Types

Yoga Principles

- ❖ Yoga promotes holistic integration of the body, mind, and spirit. It demonstrates how these aspects are interrelated and inseparable.
  - ➢ The body regulates activities, the intellect directs intelligence, and the spirit determines emotions.
  - ➢ Yoga seeks freedom (moksha) by combining the individual spirit (jeevatmaa) and universal consciousness (paramatmaa).
- ❖ **Oneness and Existence**
  - ➢ According to modern science, the cosmos is interrelated. A yogi experiences oneness and harmony with the cosmos, which transcends separateness.
- ❖ **Historical Evolution:**
  - ➢ Yoga has origins dating back over 5,000-10,000 years.
  - ➢ Early yoga scriptures were copied on delicate palm leaves.
  - ➢ Pre-Classical Yoga prioritized self-awareness, action (karma yoga), and wisdom (jnana yoga).
  - ➢ Patanjali's Yoga-Sutras describe classical yoga, which continues to be important.
  - ➢ Post-Classical Yoga embraced the physical body, resulting in Hatha Yoga.

Swami Vivekananda brought Hatha Yoga to the Western world.

<u>Types of Yoga</u>

- ❖ **Hatha Yoga**
  - ➢ Emphasizes asanas (body postures), pranayama (breathing techniques), and meditation.

- ➢ Iyengar, Integral, and Ashtanga are among the several styles.
- ❖ **Kundalini Yoga**
  - ➢ Enhances spiritual connection.
  - ➢ Includes chanting, singing, and breath-focused activities.
  - ➢ Activates Kundalini energy to promote self-awareness and spiritual enlightenment.
- ❖ **Vinyasa Yoga:** is known for its fluid sequences ("flow").
  - ➢ Allows for adjustments in speed and rest between positions.
  - ➢ Breathing is synchronized with movements.
- ❖ **Yin Yoga:**
  - ➢ Slows movements to access deep connective tissue.
  - ➢ Promotes introspection and inner discovery.
- ❖ **Bhakti Yoga:** is a form of devotional yoga.
  - ➢ Beholds the divine in everyone and everything.
  - ➢ Promotes love, compassion, and devotion.
- ❖ **Raja Yoga:** focuses on meditation and self-awareness.
  - ➢ Considered the **"King of Yoga."**

Remember that each style is tailored to various demands and preferences. Whether you want to improve your physical health, spirituality, or mental clarity, there is a yoga practice for you.

The Evolution and Popularity of Chair Yoga

Chair Yoga, an innovative modification of traditional yoga, has grown in popularity due to its accessibility and inclusiveness.

Let's look at its evolution, benefits, and techniques.

❖ **Origin and Adaptation:**

Chair Yoga was created to address the demand for more accessible yoga practices. It is designed for people who struggle to stand or get down on the floor.

> ➤ Respected instructors creatively altered basic yoga poses to be performed while sitting or utilizing a chair as support.
> ➤ The chair acts as a prop, making yoga accessible to individuals of all ages and physical levels.

❖ **Benefits:**

> ➤ Physical Benefits: Enhanced flexibility, strength, and balance.
> ➤ Increased range of motion and lower chance of injury.
> ➤ Maintaining muscle tone in people with limited mobility or chronic health issues.

❖ **Mental and emotional benefits:**

> ➤ Reducing stress, managing anxiety, and treating depression.
> ➤ Encourages calm, mindfulness, and focused breathing.
> ➤ Chair Yoga sessions promote social interaction and camaraderie.

❖ **Common Chair Yoga Poses:**

> ➤ **Seated Mountain Pose:** Improves posture and alignment by sitting on the edge of a chair with feet planted firmly.
> ➤ **Seated Cat-Cow:** A gentle spinal stretch that involves alternating between rounding and arching the spine while seated.
> ➤ **Chair Warrior:** A variant of traditional Warrior positions using a chair as support.

❖ **Scientific Research**

> ➤ **Balance Improvement:** Chair Yoga improves balance and reduces fall risk, particularly in elderly persons. A research from the University of

California, Los Angeles (UCLA) indicated that frequent Chair Yoga practice improved balance, flexibility, and strength.

❖ **Modern Context:** Chair Yoga is popular among office workers and remote professionals who spend extended periods of time seated.

➢ It promotes movement and stretching throughout the workday, counteracting the detrimental effects of extended sitting. Chair Yoga has evolved from adaptability to universal appeal, highlighting its importance in fostering physical, mental, and emotional well-being for many populations. Whether you're at home, the office, or a community class, the chair serves as a gateway to holistic wellness

Chapter 2 Understanding Chair Yoga

Chair yoga is a modified version of conventional yoga that enables you to practice while sitting. This yoga style is intended for those who may struggle with traditional poses, such as seniors, persons with mobility challenges, or those healing from injuries. Chair yoga, invented in 1982 by yoga instructor Lakshmi Voelker-Binder, employs a chair for support, assisting in balance and reducing pressure on joints such as knees and hips. Despite being soft, it is just as useful as other types of yoga. Chair yoga can be a beneficial addition to your wellness routine if you are over the age of 65, have restricted mobility, live a sedentary lifestyle, or suffer from chronic health concerns. It emphasizes remaining present, attentive breathing, and modifying positions to meet your requirements. Chair yoga helps improve balance, flexibility, and general well-being.

What Is Chair Yoga

❖ **Chair Yoga:** A Gentle Practice for All Ages and Levels

Chair yoga is a modified style of yoga in which participants practice while seated or utilizing a chair for balance.

Whether you're a novice, have mobility issues, or simply want a more accessible approach to yoga, chair yoga has several advantages.

Let's look at what chair yoga is, the benefits, and how to get started.

❖ **What is chair yoga?**

Chair yoga modifies classic yoga poses to assist persons who are unable to stand or find it difficult to move between positions.

Practitioners can execute cat/cow, warrior, sun salutations, and forward folds while seated. The fundamental premise is adaptability: start where you are, work with what you have, and do what you can. Chair yoga focuses on breath awareness, mindfulness, and self-care.

Advantages of Chair Yoga:

- ❖ **Improved Flexibility and Balance:** Consistent practice improves flexibility and balance, which are important for overall well-being.
- ❖ **Strength and Muscle Tone:** Even while seated, you can engage your core and explore joint movements to build strength.
- ❖ **Mood Enhancement:** Yoga alleviates tension, anxiety, and depression, promoting a happy attitude.
- ❖ **Better Sleep Quality:** The relaxation techniques used in chair yoga help to promote sleep.
- ❖ **Reduced Pain:** Gentle stretches reduce discomfort, making them perfect for people who have chronic diseases.
- ❖ **6. Safe Workout for Beginners:** Chair yoga promotes safety, making it appropriate for all fitness levels.
- ❖ **7. Accessible for a Wide Range of Audiences:** Chair yoga is beneficial to seniors, wheelchair users, and post-surgical patients.
- ❖ **8. Quick Workouts:** Practice chair yoga during work breaks or while traveling.

<u>**Getting Started:**</u>

- ❖ **Find a Comfortable Chair:** No specialist equipment is required; any sturdy chair without wheels will suffice.
- ❖ **Consider Your Posture:** Sit with a long spine and feet flat on the floor. If your feet cannot reach, use blocks or a folded mat.
- ❖ **Breathing Techniques:** Align motions with your breath—inhale during expansion and exhale during contraction.
- ❖ **Example Poses:**
  - ➢ **Chair Cat-Cow Stretch:** Sit tall, inhale arching your back (cow), exhale rounding (cat).

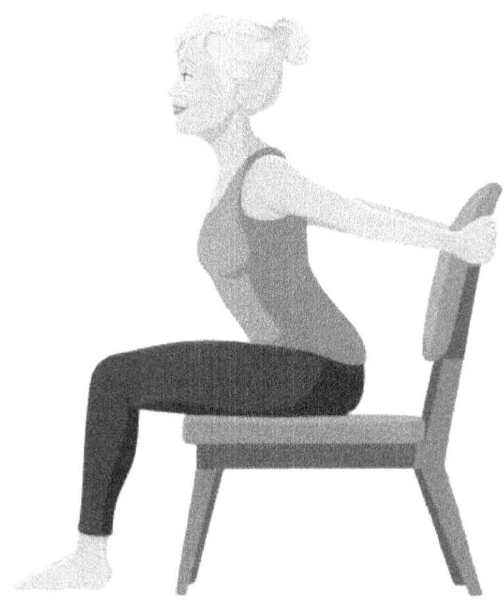

> **Seated Forward Bend:** Hinge at the hips and extend towards your feet.

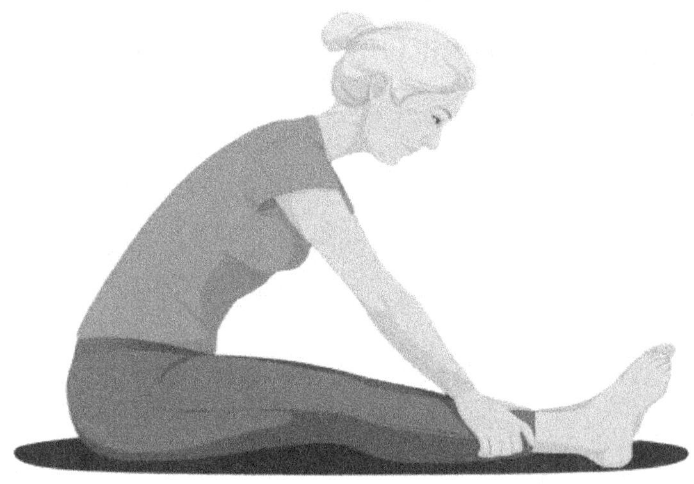

> **Seated Eagle Pose:** Cross arms at elbows and raise hands to the ceiling.

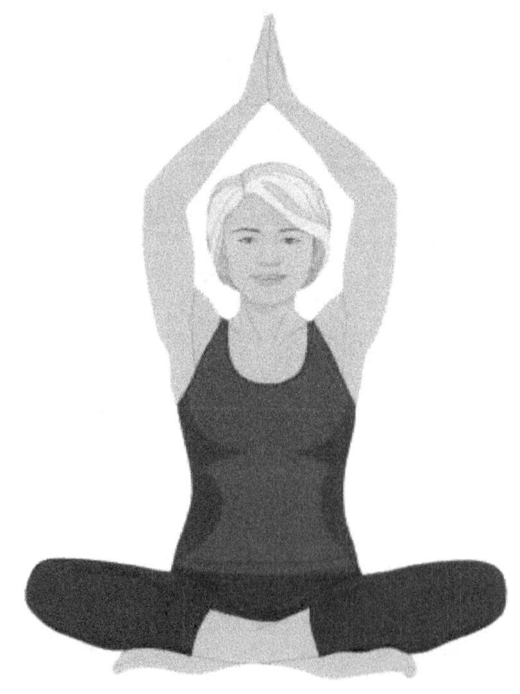

➢ **Seated Twist:** Rotate your torso gently while looking over one shoulder.

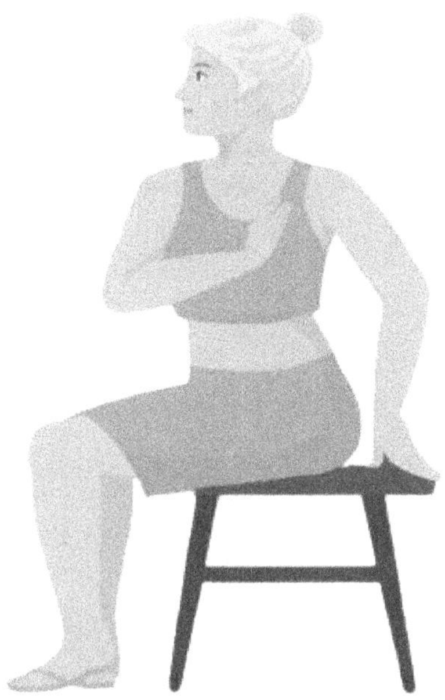

➢ **Chair Pigeon Pose:** Cross one ankle over the opposing knee while remaining upright.

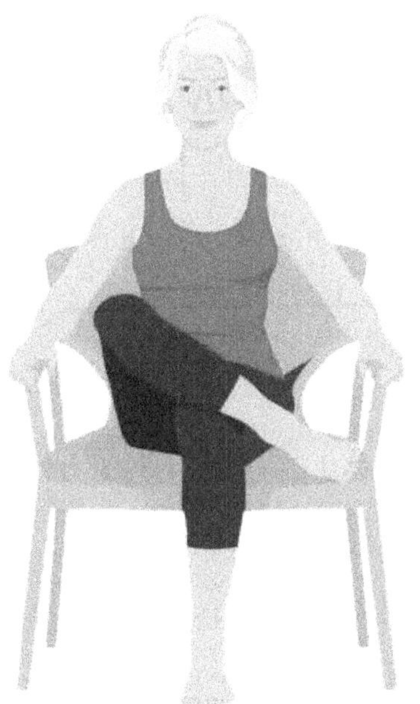

> **Seated Chest Opener:** Place your hands behind your back, raise your chest, and open your heart.

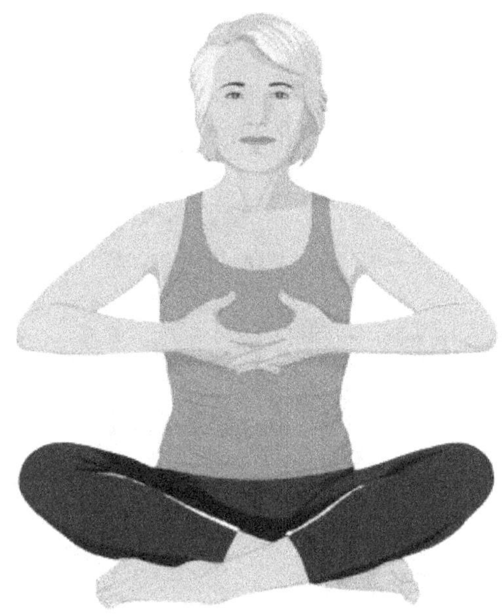

* ❖ **Practice Mindfully.** Pay attention to sensations, make adjustments as appropriate, and respect your body's boundaries.

Remember that chair yoga isn't about perfecting poses; it's about improving your overall health. Whether you're at home, work, or a community class, accept flexibility and enjoy the adventure!

Benefits of Chair Yoga for Seniors Over 60

Chair yoga is a great approach for adults over 60 to maintain and improve their physical health, flexibility, and mental well-being. This yoga style allows for seated or chair-supported poses, making it suitable for persons with restricted mobility or beginners.

<u>**Below are several significant advantages:**</u>

- ❖ **Improved Strength:** Chair yoga strengthens muscles in the upper body, core, and legs. It focuses on muscle areas that are necessary for daily actions such as standing, reaching, and lifting objects.

- ❖ **Enhanced Flexibility:** Chair yoga improves joint mobility and flexibility. Seniors can gently stretch their muscles without placing too much strain on their joints.

- ❖ **Better equilibrium:** As we become older, it becomes increasingly important to keep our equilibrium. Chair yoga emphasizes stability and coordination, which helps seniors improve their balance and lower their chance of falling.

- ❖ **Reduced Stress:** Mindfulness and relaxation techniques used in chair yoga boost mental health. Seniors can relieve stress, anxiety, and tension with moderate movements and breathing exercises.

- ❖ **Community Connection:** Chair yoga classes foster a sense of community. Seniors can mingle, share their experiences, and form connections with others in a supportive setting

- ❖ **Low-Impact Exercise:** Chair yoga is soft on the joints and appropriate for people with arthritis or other health issues. It enables elders to remain active without placing pressure on their bodies.

- ❖ **Increased Energy:** Regular exercise improves circulation, oxygenates the body, and energizes elders. It reduces weariness and increases overall energy.

- ❖ **Better Posture:** Chair yoga promotes optimal alignment and awareness of body posture. Seniors learn how to sit and stand with proper spinal alignment.

- ❖ **Mind-Body Connection:** Yoga promotes a stronger connection between the mind and body. Seniors may feel less discomfort, better sleep, and greater self-awareness.
- ❖ **Accessible and Inclusive:** Chair yoga can be practiced anywhere, whether at home, a community center, or at work. Seniors can take part regardless of their fitness level or physical constraints.
- ❖ **Breathing Exercises:** Chair yoga uses attentive breathing methods. Seniors learn to breathe deeply, which reduces stress and promotes relaxation.
- ❖ **Better Sleep:** Seniors who do chair yoga frequently report better sleep quality. Yoga's soothing effects improve sleep quality

Chair yoga offers a comprehensive approach to well-being that incorporates physical activity, mental focus, and community involvement. Seniors can reap the advantages of yoga without the need for complicated positions or strenuous physical activity. Chair yoga, whether done at home or in a group setting, helps seniors stay healthy and active.

Chair Yoga vs. Traditional Yoga

Let's look at the differences between chair yoga and traditional yoga.

- ❖ **Definition and Approach:**
  - ➢ **Chair Yoga:** Traditional yoga poses are modified to be performed while sitting or utilizing a chair as support. It is suitable for people with limited movement, elders, and those recovering from injuries.

- ➢ **Traditional yoga:** Traditional yoga consists of physical poses (asanas), meditation (dyana), and breathing exercises (pranayama). It is often done on a mat, with standing, seated, and lying-down poses.

- ❖ **Physical Poses:**
  - ➢ **Chair Yoga:** Poses are modified to fit sitting or utilizing a chair for balance. A modified downward dog can be performed by placing hands on the chair seat.
  - ➢ **Traditional Yoga:** Traditional yoga includes a variety of poses such as standing, balancing, twisting, and inversion.
- ❖ **Intensity and Calorie Burn:**
  - ➢ **Chair Yoga:** A low-impact exercise that promotes flexibility, balance, and relaxation. The calorie burn is rather minimal compared to more strenuous pursuits.
  - ➢ **Traditional Yoga** The intensity varies, ranging from moderate Hatha yoga to rigorous Vinyasa or Ashtanga. The dynamic movements provide a larger calorie burn.
- ❖ **Accessibility:**
  - ➢ **Chair Yoga:** Suitable for elders, individuals with mobility challenges, and novices. Creates a safe and supportive environment.
  - ➢ **Traditional yoga:** Suitable for a wide spectrum of practitioners, although may be difficult for some owing to physical requirements.
- ❖ **Equipment:**
  - ➢ **Chair Yoga:** Use a solid chair made for yoga practice.
  - ➢ **Traditional Yoga:** Typically performed on a yoga mat, with optional supports such as blocks and straps.
  - ➢

- ❖ **Benefits:**
  - ➢ **Chair Yoga:** Enhances strength, flexibility, balance, and mental health. Reduces stress and fosters communal connections.
  - ➢ **Traditional Yoga:** Provides similar benefits, but focuses on spiritual growth and self-awareness.
- ❖ **Breathing Techniques:**
  - ➢ **Chair Yoga:** Uses focused breathing exercises to relieve stress and promote relaxation.
  - ➢ **Traditional Yoga:** Pranayama methods are essential for traditional yoga and promote overall well-being.
- ❖ **Community and Social Aspect:**
  - ➢ **Chair Yoga:** Classes foster a sense of belonging and support.
  - ➢ **Traditional Yoga:** Typically practiced in group settings to develop bonds.
- ❖ **Mind-Body Connection:**
  - ➢ **Chair Yoga:** Increases awareness of body and breath.
  - ➢ **Traditional Yoga:** Improves the mind-body connection via meditation and awareness.

Chair yoga provides a mild, accessible approach, whereas conventional yoga includes a wider range of poses and activities.

Both have distinct advantages, and the choice is based on personal preferences, needs, and physical abilities.

Chapter 3: Preparing for Chair Yoga

Chair yoga is a moderate style of yoga that can be performed while sitting on a chair or standing with a chair as support.

How to Prepare for Chair Yoga:

- ❖ **Choose the Right Chair:** Choose a robust chair with no wheels. Sit with your feet level on the floor and knees at a 90-degree angle.
- ❖ **Wear Comfortable clothes:** Choose loose, comfortable clothes that allows for easy movement.
- ❖ **Create a Safe Space:** Choose a calm, distraction-free location. To avoid slippage, place the chair on a solid surface such as a yoga mat or carpet.
- ❖ **Begin with Breathing Exercises:** Each session should start with a few minutes of deep breathing to center yourself.
- ❖ Warm up with simple stretches for neck, shoulders, back, and ankles.
- ❖ **Progress to Yoga positions:** Practice fundamental sitting positions such as Mountain Pose and Forward Bending. Gradually on to more intermediate and advanced poses as you feel comfortable.

Remember that chair yoga is adjustable and appropriate for all ages and abilities. Enjoy the benefits of yoga without the need for a mat or much floor work!

Building the Right Mindset for Yoga Practice

Developing the correct mindset for a meaningful yoga practice is critical for both new and experienced practitioners.

<u>Below are '12 mentality shifts' to improve your yoga journey:</u>

- ❖ **Begin Small:** If you're new to yoga or returning from a break, start with short practice sessions. Gradually increase the duration as you develop consistency. Remember that developing a new habit takes time.

- ❖ **Minutes Is Enough:** Recognize that even a brief practice is important. Five minutes of mindful movement or breathing exercises can be profound. Prioritize self-care and self-love, rather than harsh expectations.

- ❖ **Make Decisions in Advance:** Schedule your practice ahead of time to show your commitment. Set intentions and treat your mat time like a gift to yourself. Avoid last-minute decisions that result in skipping practice.

- ❖ **Your Practice and Rules:** Release the urge to meet external norms. Your practice is individual. Change up your poses, experiment with different variants, and listen to your body. Focus on your well-being rather than perfection.

- ❖ **Listen In and Develop** inward awareness. Pay attention to your body's sensations, breath, and thoughts. Yoga is a discussion with oneself. Pay attention and make any adjustments.

- ❖ **Know Your Limits:** Maintain your physical and mental boundaries. Yoga is not about pushing through pain. Respect your current situation and make incremental development. Compassion for yourself is essential.

- ❖ **Give Yourself A Break:** Life happens. Missed practices and unsatisfactory sessions are typical. Instead of criticizing yourself, be gentle. Celebrate showing up, even if it's not perfect.

- ❖ **Embrace the Suck:** Some days, practice is difficult. Embrace discomfort; it is where progress occurs. Accept that not every session will be pleasant, and that's fine.
- ❖ **Cultivate a Positive Mindset:** Practice meditation, affirmations, and gratitude. An optimistic mindset increases motivation and well-being. Join a supportive community, in-person or online.
- ❖ **Challenge Limiting Beliefs:** Replace self-doubt with positive thoughts. Believe in your own abilities to improve. Yoga promotes transformation, both physically and mentally.
- ❖ **Practice Mindfulness:** Stay present on your mat. Let go of distractions and judgment. Every breath, every movement counts. Mindfulness improves the quality of your practice.
- ❖ **Be Patient and Persistent:** Progress does not happen overnight. Trust in the process. Consistency is more important than occasional intensity. Celebrate minor achievements and remain devoted to your practice. Do not forget that your yoga practice is a continuous journey. Cultivate a mindset of self-compassion, curiosity, and growth.
- ❖

Overcoming Common Obstacles to Starting Yoga

Overcoming barriers in yoga practice is critical for development and advancement. **<u>Let's look at some frequent challenges and ways to solve them:</u>**

- ❖ **Health Concerns:** Physical and mental health issues might impede yoga practice. It is critical to tailor poses and sequences to each individual's demands. Consult a healthcare professional as needed.
- ❖ **Apathy:** Are you unmotivated to practice? Set small, manageable goals and seek inspiration from yoga communities, teachers, or internet platforms.

- ❖ **Self-Doubt:** Do you doubt your own abilities? Always remember that yoga is a journey, not a destination. Focus on the process and recognize minor successes.
- ❖ **Carelessness:** Consistency is crucial. Avoid skipping practice sessions. Practice mindfulness and stick to your routine.
- ❖ **Distractions:** During practice, identify all distractions (internal and external). Create a specific space, disable notifications, and stay present.
- ❖ **Misplaced Priorities:** Schedule time for yoga. Prioritize self-care and well-being. Even brief sessions can be effective.
- ❖ **Physical Illness:** If you are ill, adjust your practice. Gentle stretches and restorative poses can assist. Listen to your body.
- ❖ **Cravings:** Control your food cravings. Make nourishing choices that support your practice. Stay hydrated and avoid heavy meals before yoga.
- ❖ **Egoism:** Let go of self-imposed expectations. Yoga is to promote self-discovery and growth, not perfection.

Mind you perseverance, patience, and continuous practice contribute to progress. Embrace the trip and reap the benefits of chair yoga for seniors over 60!

Tips for Practicing Chair Yoga Safely

When practicing chair yoga, safety comes first.

<u>Below are some crucial guidelines to always keep in mind:</u>

- ❖ **Listen to Your Body:** If a position causes pain or discomfort, stop right away. Trust your body's signals.
- ❖ **Use Props:** Blocks and blankets can help you feel more comfortable and change up your stances. They offer support and stability.

- ❖ **Practice Regularly:** Consistency is essential for reaping the advantages of chair yoga. Make it part of your routine.

Remember that chair yoga is adjustable and appropriate for a variety of age groups, including seniors and office professionals. Enjoy your practice

Things to Avoid in Chair Yoga

Below are some crucial things to avoid while practicing chair yoga.

- ❖ **To avoid slouching or hunching over**: keep your back upright and your shoulders relaxed. Slumping can strain the spine and muscles.
- ❖ **Ignoring Breath Awareness:** Remember that breathing is essential to yoga. Practice mindful breathing during poses.
- ❖ **Overstretching:** Avoid forcing oneself into uncomfortable positions. Allow yourself to move at your own pace.
- ❖ **Using Unstable Chairs:** Select a solid chair with a flat seat and backrest. Avoid chairs with arms or wheels that limit movement.
- ❖ **Incorrect Posture and Alignment:** Pay attention to your alignment. Proper posture helps prevent strain and injury.

Remember that chair yoga emphasizes gentle movement and self-care.

How to Create a Chair Yoga Practice at Home

Developing a chair yoga practice at home is an excellent method to improve flexibility, reduce stress, and boost general health.

Below are guide to get you started:

- ❖ **Choose a Sturdy Chair** with a Flat Seat and Backrest. Avoid chairs with wheels or arms that limit mobility.
  - ➤ If your feet don't reach the floor, place blocks or a folded yoga mat beneath them to provide a solid platform.
- ❖ **Set Up Your Space:**
  - ➤ Choose a quiet, comfortable environment with little distractions.
  - ➤ Arrange items that inspire you, such as a quiet candle or relaxing music.
- ❖ **Begin with Breathing Exercises:** Begin each session with a few minutes of deep breathing. Practice slow and attentive breathing. This helps to focus your attention and prepares you for the practice.
  - ❖ **Warm up with simple stretches:** such as head circles, shoulder shrugs, and torso stretches.
  - ➤ These movements enhance circulation and flexibility.
- ❖ **Progress to Yoga positions:**
  - ➤ Practice adapted yoga positions while sitting.
  - ➤ **Chair Cat-Cow Stretch:** Sit tall and place both feet on the floor. Inhale, arch your back (cow), and exhale by rounding your spine (cat).

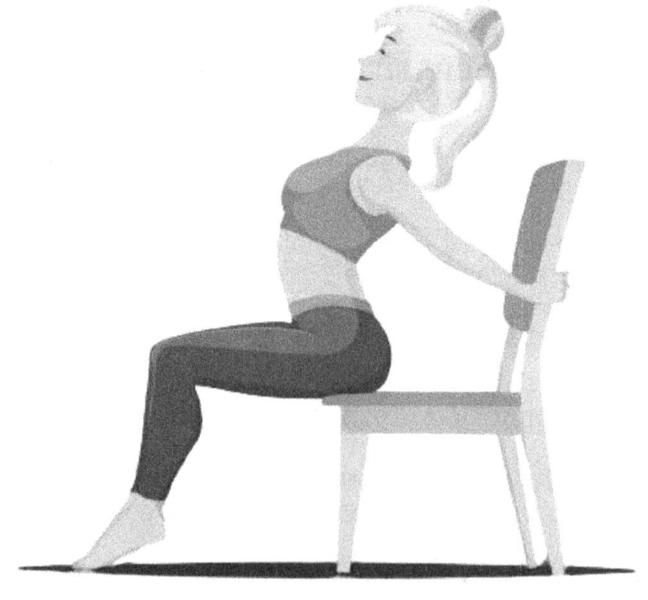

➢ **Mountain Pose:** Sit straight with your feet grounded and raise your arms high.

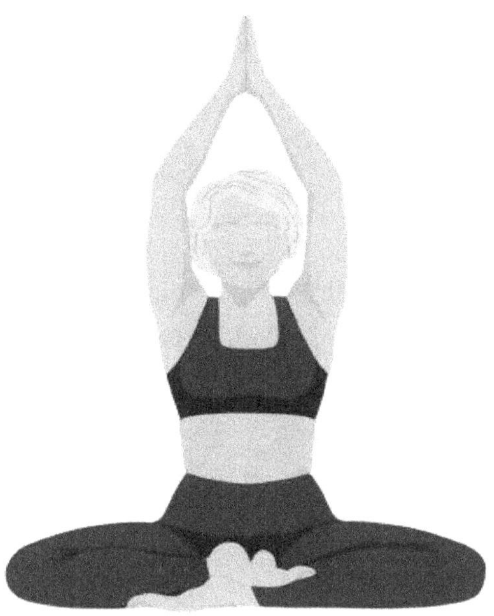

➢ **Staff Pose:** Extend your legs forward, flex your feet, and stretch your spine.

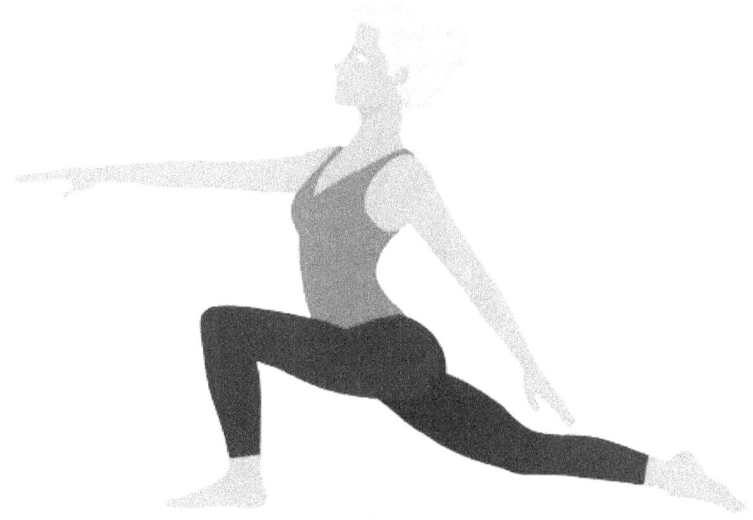

➢ **Goddess Pose:** Spread your knees wide while maintaining your feet flat on the ground.

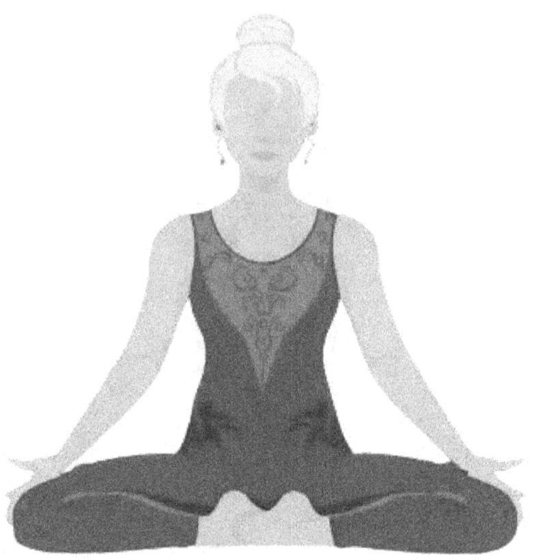

➢ **Spinal Twist:** Twist gently to each side while supporting with your hands.

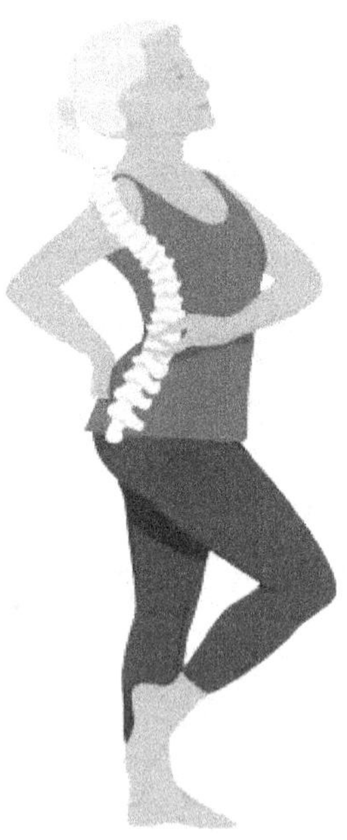

➢ **Hip Opener:** Place one ankle over the opposing knee and gently press down.

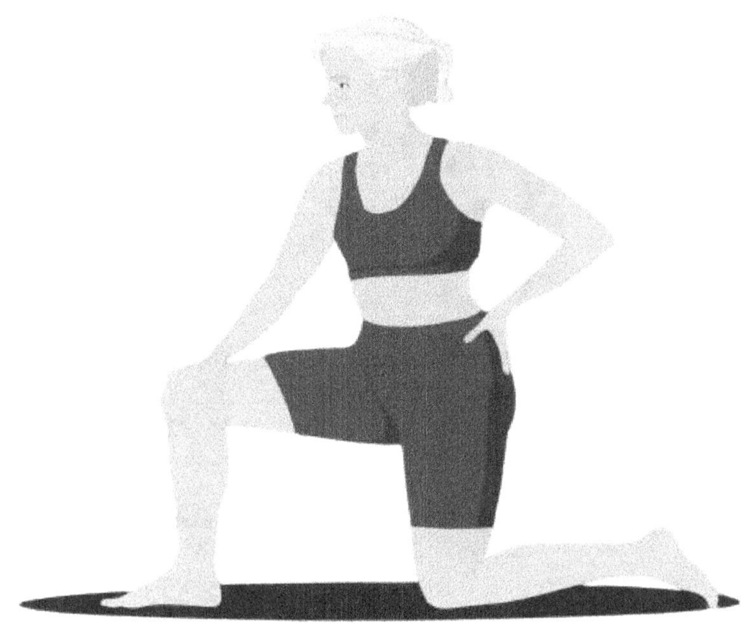

➢ **Side Bend:** Reach one arm above and lean to the other side.

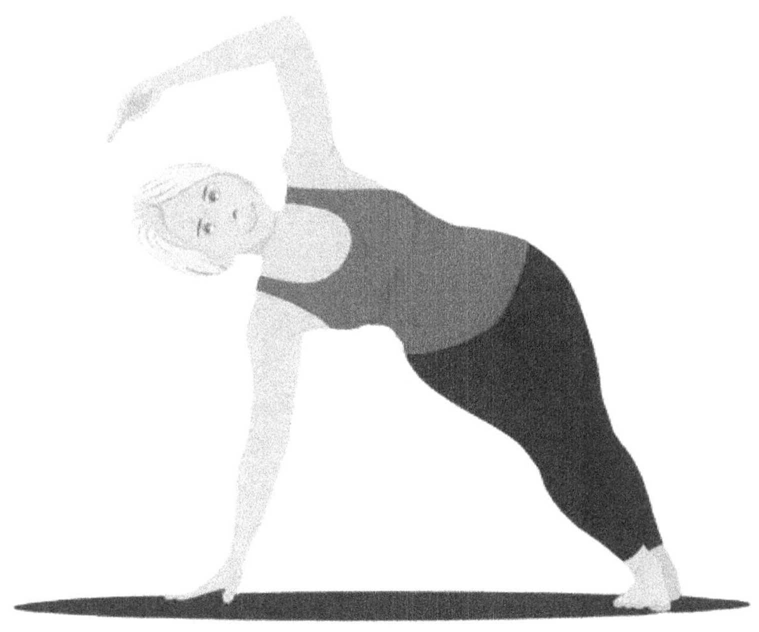

➢ **Half Forward Bend:** Hinge at the hips and stretch toward your feet.

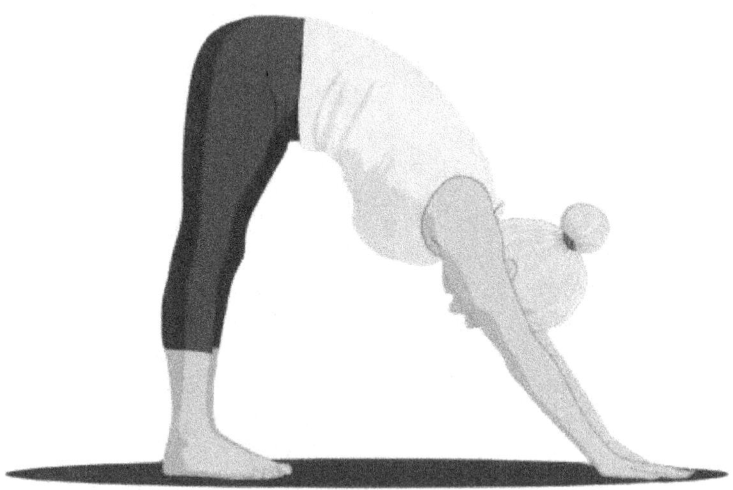

❖ **Chest Opener:** Place your hands behind your back and raise your chest.

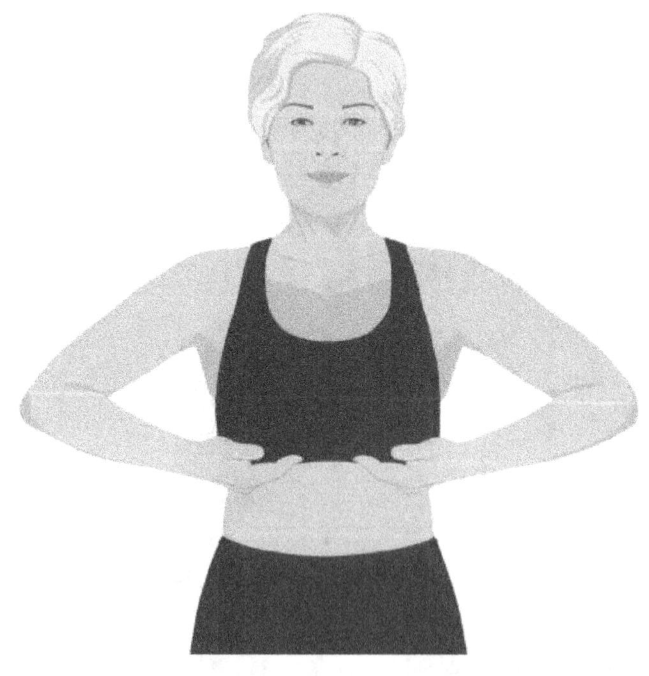

➢ **Torso Stretch:** Raise both arms and lean to one side.

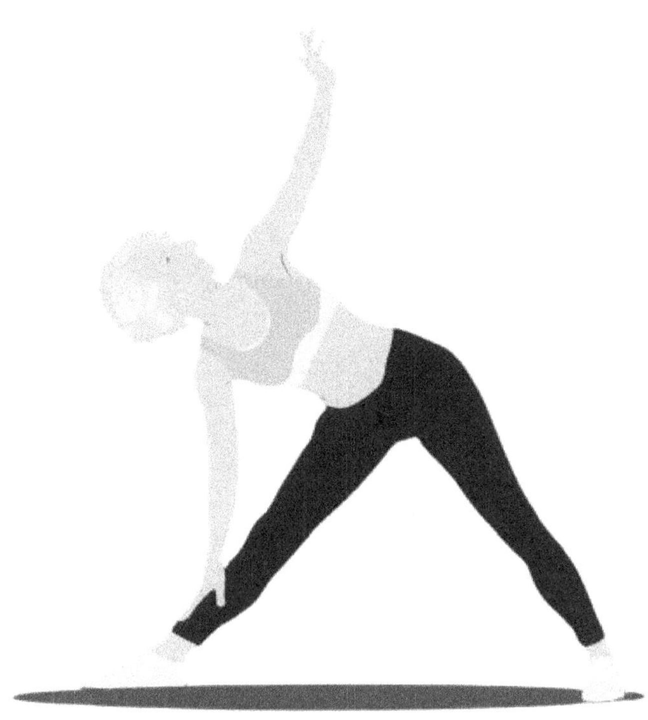

❖ **Use Props as Needed:**

➢ Modify positions with pillows, belts, or towels for support.

➢ Adapt the practice to your state of ease and contentment.

❖ **End with Relaxation:** Conclude your session with a few minutes of relaxation.

➢ Close your eyes, relax, and release any stress.

❖ **Practice consistently**. Aim for brief sessions each day or lengthier practices a few times per week.

➢ give attention to your body and make any necessary corrections. Recall that chair yoga is adaptive and accessible to everybody. Whether you're recovering from an injury, require additional assistance, or simply want a therapeutic approach, you may get the benefits of yoga from the comfort of your chair!

Chapter 4: Breathing and Warm-Up Techniques

Breathing methods are important in chair yoga because they promote relaxation, focus, and overall well-being. Here are a few crucial practices:

- ❖ **Deep Breathing:** Start by sitting comfortably in your chair.
  - ➢ Rest your palms on your thighs. Inhale fully, then exhale completely.
  - ➢ You can breathe in and out of either your nose or your mouth.
  - ➢ Aim for a complete circle from inhalation to exhalation.
  - ➢ Repeat the cycle 30-40 times.
  - ➢ After the final round, try to hold your breath for as long as possible.
- ❖ **Ujjayi Breathing:** This practice balances and relaxes the body. Inhale deeply via your nose, slightly tightening the back of your throat. Exhale slowly via your nose, making a smooth ocean-like sound. It reduces tension and improves focus.
- ❖ **Kapalbhati:** A cleaning breath that involves exhaling forcefully through the nostrils while inhaling passively. It cleanses the respiratory system and revitalizes the body.
- ❖ **Alternate Nostril Breathing:** Sit comfortably, then use your thumb and ring finger to seal one nostril at a time. Inhale through one nostril and then switch to exhale through the other. This activity encourages relaxation and balance.

❖ **Viloma:** teaches us to breathe more deeply. Inhale in quick bursts, pausing between each one. Exhale easily. This approach increases lung capacity and promotes attentive breathing.

<u>For 'warm-up' try mild motions to prepare your body:</u>

❖ **Seated Side Bends:** Sit upright, inhale, and raise one arm overhead. Exhale and bend sideways. Repeat on the opposite side.

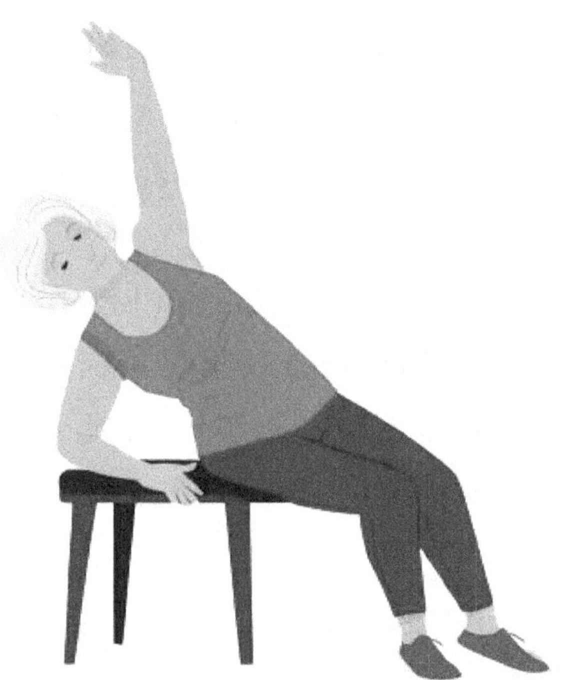

❖ **Seated Twists:** Inhale, stretch your spine, then gently twist to one side. Exhale and twist to the other side.

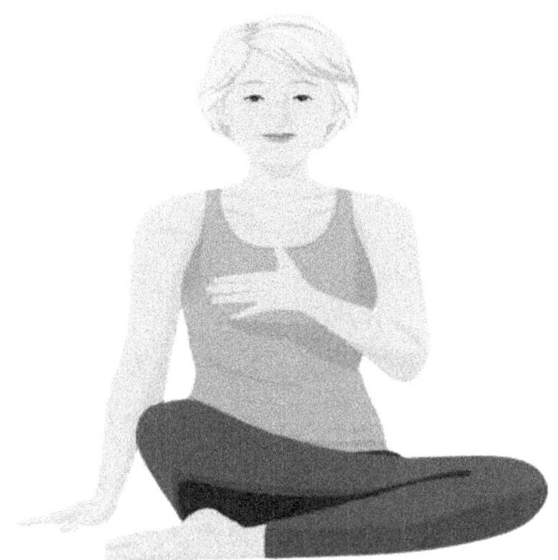

❖ **Shoulder Circles:** Roll your shoulders forwards and backwards to relieve tension.

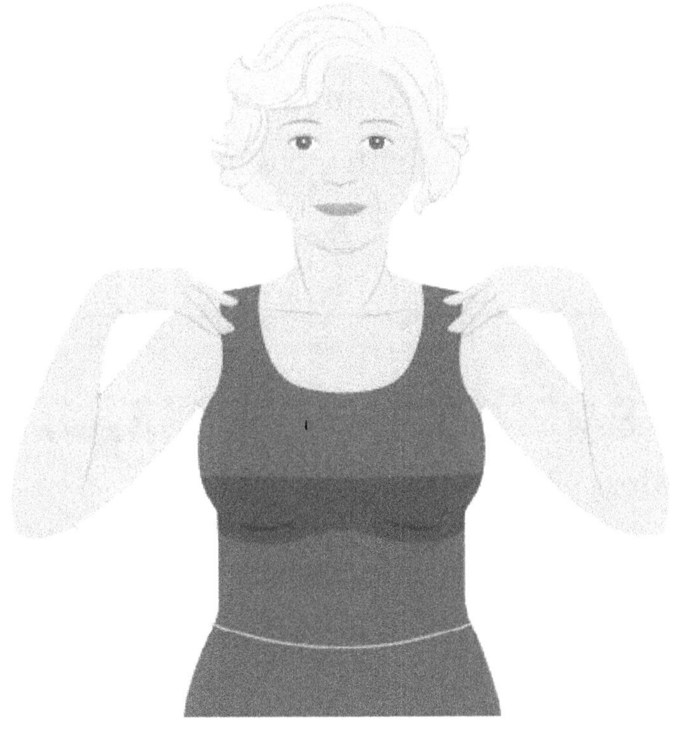

❖ **Wrist Stretches:** stretch your arms, flex and stretch your wrists, then spin them in both directions.

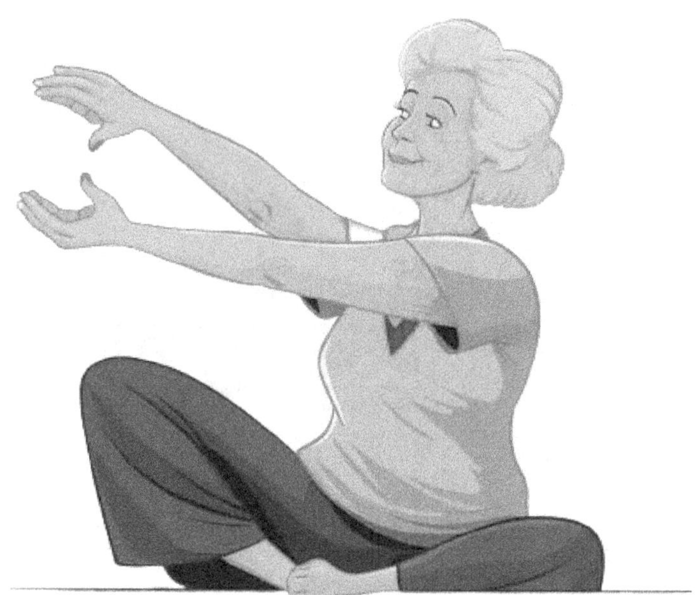

Remember to ask your doctor before beginning any exercise program. Chair yoga is an excellent way to keep active, enhance circulation, and preserve flexibility, particularly for seniors.

The Importance of Breath in Yoga

The importance of breath in yoga cannot be emphasized.

<u>Let's look at how it dramatically affects our practice:</u>

- ❖ **Biologically:** Focusing on our breath during asana practice transfers control from the brain stem to the cerebral cortex.
    - ➢ This awareness produces magic
    - ➢ The mind grows quieter, and calmness emerges.
    - ➢ Emotionally, this eliminates tension and wandering thoughts, letting energy (prana) to flow freely, unclogging the body and mind.

This connection is responsible for the "feel-good" sensation following yoga practice.

- ❖ **Physically:** Breath awareness affects structural alignment. It prevents joint compression and imbalances in postures. Ashtanga Vinyasa[1] relies on fluid movement as its base.
- ❖ **Mind and Breath:** There is a strong relationship between the breath and mind. The change in breath indicates mental alterations.
    - ➢ Mindfulness of breathing leads to insight into the nature of the mind, ultimately liberating us from pain.
    - ➢ Freedom from suffering is not the same as freedom from pain; it's about how we deal with pain and let go.

Breath is the vital force that connects mind, body, and spirit in yoga. Each inhalation and exhalation energizes, soothes, and strengthens our mind-body connection.

Chair Yoga Breathing Exercises

'Chair yoga breathing exercises' are a gentle yet effective technique to improve overall well-being, reduce stress, and encourage relaxation.

Let's look at some essential aspects:

- ❖ **Mindful Breathing:** In chair yoga, we emphasize aware breathing.
  - ➢ Encourage seniors to sit comfortably, with their spines aligned and their feet anchored.
  - ➢ Invite them to breathe deeply through their nose, expanding their abdomen, and then gently exhale through pursed lips.

Taking thoughtful breaths can relax the nervous system and promote the "rest and digest" response.

- ❖ **Ujjayi Breath:** Also known as the **"ocean breath,"** ujjayi involves slightly narrowing the throat on both inhalation and exhale. It warms up the body, relaxes the mind, and increases lung capacity. Seniors can practice ujjayi while sitting, experiencing a calm ocean-like sound in their throat.
- ❖ **Alternate Nostril Breathing:** This practice rebalances energy channels. Inhale through one nostril, close it with your thumb, then exhale through the other. Then flip sides. It balances the neurological system, decreases anxiety, and enhances focus.
- ❖ **Deep Belly Breathing:** Encourage seniors to rest their hands on their abdomens. The belly expands as they inhale and collapses when they exhale. Deep belly breathing promotes tissue oxygenation, mental relaxation, and digestion.
- ❖ **Sitali Breath:** Roll the tongue into a **"U"** shape and breathe through it. Exhale via your nose. Sitali cools the body, lowers stress, and improves lung function. Seniors can practice comfortably on a chair.
- ❖ **Kumbhaka (Breath Retention):** After taking a full intake, wait briefly before exhalation. This increases lung capacity, sharpens focus, and energizes the body. Seniors should begin with shorter holds and gradually increase duration.

Remember that chair yoga breathing exercises are adjustable. Seniors can practice them anywhere, including at home, work, and during breaks. Encourage consistency, and these basic habits will benefit their general well-being

Chair Yoga Warm-Up Exercises and Stretches

Chair yoga warm-up movements and stretches are critical for preparing the body, increasing flexibility, and encouraging calm. Let's look at some successful warm-up routines:

- ❖ **Neck Stretches:** Slowly tilt your head towards each shoulder and hold for a few breaths. This helps to relieve stress in the neck and upper back.
- ❖ **Shoulder Rolls:**
  - ➤ Circularly move your shoulders forth and backward. This warms the shoulder joints and increases mobility.
- ❖ **Wrist Stretches:**
  - ➤ Extend your arms forward and flex your wrists up/down. This helps to preserve wrist flexibility and prevent stiffness.
- ❖ **Cat/Cow Movements:**
  - ➤ Sit tall in your chair, hands on thighs.
  - ➤ Inhale, arch your spine (like a cat), and raise your chest and chin.
  - ➤ Exhale, round your spine (like a cow), and tuck your chin to your chest.
  - ➤ Repeat the gentle spinal movement many times.
- ❖ **Sun Salutation Arm Movements:** Extend arms aloft with palms facing each other.
  - ➤ Inhale, reach up, and extend your spine.
  - ➤ Exhale and lower your arms back down.
  - ➤ Repeat this flow several times to stimulate your upper body.

- ❖ **Forward Folds:**
  - ➤ Sit on the edge of your chair, feet hip-width apart.
  - ➤ Inhale, stretch your spine, and exhale as you bend forward from your hips.
  - ➤ Bring your hands to the floor or your shins.
  - ➤ Take deep breaths and feel the stretch in your hamstrings and lower back
- ❖ **Twists:**
  - ➤ Sit sideways in your chair and hold the backrest.
  - ➤ Inhale, stretch your spine, then exhale as you twist to one side.
  - ➤ Hold for a few breaths before switching to the opposite side.
  - ➤ Twists increase spinal mobility and assist digestion.
- ❖ **Side Bends:**
  - ➤ Sit tall and extend one arm above.
  - ➤ Gently bend to the opposite side and feel the stretch along your ribcage.
  - ➤ Repeat on the opposite side.

Not forget to breathe deeply throughout these warm-up activities. They not only prepare your body for more strenuous activities, but also encourage relaxation and overall well-being. As usual, contact with your doctor before beginning any workout regimen.

Chapter 5: Chair Yoga for Health and Wellness

Chair yoga is a moderate and accessible style of yoga that can greatly improve overall health and wellness. Whether you're a senior, have restricted mobility, or simply want a more pleasant practice, chair yoga has several advantages.

- ❖ **Physical Benefits:**
- ❖ **Flexibility and Mobility:** Chair yoga promotes joint flexibility by stretching muscles and increasing range of motion. It is especially good for elders who may have stiffness or limited mobility.
- ❖ **Strength Building:** Seated postures work several muscular groups, such as the core, arms, and legs. Regular practice can help improve muscle tone and stability.
- ❖ **Improved Posture:** Chair yoga promotes appropriate alignment, which helps reduce back discomfort and improve posture.
- ❖ **Circulation and Breathing:** Gentle movements increase blood flow and deep breathing, which improves oxygen intake and promotes relaxation.
- ❖ **Mental and Emotional Well-Being:**
- ❖ **Tension Reduction:** Chair yoga incorporates mindful breathing and relaxation techniques to alleviate tension and anxiety. Focusing on the current moment promotes a state of tranquility.
- ❖ **Mind-Body Connection:** Chair yoga promotes awareness by allowing practitioners to connect with their own bodies and sensations. This understanding encourages self-acceptance and care.

- ❖ **Increased Concentration:** The combination of movement and breathing promotes mental clarity and focus.
- ❖ **Social Interaction:** Group chair yoga lessons offer social support and help people overcome feelings of isolation.
- ❖ **Safety considerations**
- ❖ **Individualized Practice:** Chair yoga can be tailored to each person's requirements and skills. Consult with a trained instructor about tailoring the practice to your individual needs.
- ❖ **Avoid Overexertion:** Listen to your body and don't push yourself too much. The idea is gradual movement, not strenuous exertion.
- ❖ **Breathing Awareness:** Pay attention to your breath when in positions. Slow, deep breaths promote relaxation and oxygenation in the body.

Remember that chair yoga is more than simply physical poses; it is a whole practice that benefits both body and mind. Whether you're at home, work, or a community center, including chair yoga into your routine can help you feel better and have more energy.

Chair Yoga for Physical Health: Flexibility, Strength, and Balance

Below is a quick guide to Chair Yoga for Physical Health: Flexibility, Strength, and Balance:

- ❖ **Improved Flexibility and Mobility:** Regular practice gently stretches and strengthens the body, increasing flexibility and joint mobility.
  - ➤ The adjusted poses target specific muscle areas, increasing suppleness and preventing stiffness.

- Improved flexibility leads to a wider range of motion and greater ease of daily activities.
- ❖ **Improved Strength and Balance:**
  - ➢ Chair yoga promotes strength in multiple areas.
  - ➢ **Upper Body:** Poses that work the arms, shoulders, and chest.
  - ➢ **Core:** Strengthening the core muscles improves stability and balance.
  - ➢ **Lower Body:** Leg lifts and ankle exercises increase lower-body strength. Better balance minimizes the chance of falls, which is especially important for elderly.
  - ➢ Stronger muscles facilitate daily chores and increase coordination
- ❖ **Posture and Alignment:** Practicing chair yoga improves posture.
  - ➢ Proper alignment decreases strain on the spine and back discomfort.
  - ➢ Good posture improves general well-being.
- ❖ **Mind-Body Connection:**
  - ➢ Mindful breathing and focused movements promote tranquility.
  - ➢ Chair yoga improves mental clarity while reducing stress and anxiety.
  - ➢ Participants connect with their bodies, which increases self-awareness.
- ❖ **Adaptability and Accessibility:**
  - ➢ Chair yoga can be practiced anywhere, including offices, homes, and community centers.
  - ➢ It can suit a wide range of fitness levels and physical problems.
  - ➢ Modifications enable everyone to engage, regardless of constraints.
- ❖ **Sample Chair Yoga Routine (13 minutes):**
  - ➢ Begin with seated deep breaths to ground oneself.
  - ➢ Warm up by lifting heels and performing squats with chair support.
  - ➢ Practice balancing on one leg, tapping toes, and stretching the leg backward.

- ➤ Use the chair to practice yoga positions such as **"airplane"** and **"tree".**
- ➤ For an added challenge, perform arm circles while holding your arms out.
- ➤ Cool down by marching with elevated knees before returning to your chair. Remember to ask your doctor before beginning any exercise program. Chair yoga is a gentle, accessible way to improve physical health, flexibility, and overall well-being. Enjoy your practice!

Chair Yoga for Mental Health, Stress Relief and Mindfulness

Chair yoga is a peaceful and accessible yoga style in which participants execute poses while seated in chairs. It focuses on mindfulness, deep breathing, and gentle movements.

<u>Below is why chair yoga is good for your mental health, stress reduction, and mindfulness:</u>

Chair yoga is accessible and inclusive to people of all ages, including seniors, those with mobility challenges, and those with impairments.

- ➤ It offers physical support, boosts confidence, and promotes a sense of community.
- ❖ **Stress Reduction:** Chair yoga, like conventional yoga, focuses on deep breathing and mindfulness methods. Sitting relaxation techniques enhance calm, reduce stress, and improve emotional well-being.
- ❖ **Mindfulness and Clarity:**
  - ➤ Focusing on movement, breath, and bodily reactions leads to a moving meditation.
  - ➤ It increases mental clarity, lowers tension, and promotes relaxation.

➢ Seated yoga may also help reduce anxiety and despair.

❖ **Simple Practices:** Easily incorporate chair yoga into your regular practice.

➢ Sit down and try wrist stretches, neck rolls, twists, or easy Sun breaths.

In conclusion, chair yoga provides a comprehensive approach to wellness, combining physical advantages with mental and emotional support. Whether you're a beginner or an experienced yogi, chair yoga can provide a peaceful and stress-relieving practice.

Chair Yoga for Specific Conditions and Injuries

Chair yoga is a modified version of traditional yoga created primarily for elders and people with mobility issues. It provides several benefits without requiring a yoga mat or difficult poses.

Let's look into chair yoga for specific diseases and injuries:

❖ **Benefits of Chair Yoga:**

➢ **Improves Flexibility and Mobility:** Gentle stretches and motions support seniors' range of motion.

➢ **Improves Balance and Stability:** Poses promote balance, lowering the danger of falling.

➢ **Reduces Stress and Promotes Relaxation:** Mindful breathing and meditation are relaxing practices.

❖ **Targeted Poses for Specific Conditions:**

❖ **Arthritis:** Chair yoga can help relieve symptoms by gently moving joints and increasing circulation.

❖ **Balance Issues:** Poses that improve stability are helpful in fall prevention.

- ❖ **Chronic Pain:** Gentle motions can ease muscle tightness and discomfort.
- ❖ **Getting Started with Chair Yoga:**
  - ➢ **Selecting a Suitable Chair:** Choose a stable chair without wheels for proper back support.
  - ➢ **Warm up Exercises:** Before beginning the main routine, perform some easy neck rotations, shoulder rolls, and ankle circles.
- ❖ **Safety Precautions:**
  - ➢ **Adapt Exercises:** Modify positions based on fitness level and personal needs.
  - ➢ **Ask a healthcare professional:** Seek counsel before beginning chair yoga.
- ❖ **Success Stories and Mental Health Benefits:** Consistent chair yoga practice has led to enhanced well-being for many seniors. Mindful breathing has relaxing effects that can help with anxiety and sleeplessness. To summarize, chair yoga is a gentle yet effective way to keep active, increase flexibility, and address specific health conditions. Always remember to consult a professional to reap the benefits of this simple procedure!

Chapter 6: Beginner Chair Yoga Practices

Let's look at the fundamental techniques of chair yoga for beginners.

Chair yoga is a gentle and accessible style of yoga that allows seniors over 60 to reap the benefits of yoga without having to lie down on the floor. It's a wonderful technique to increase your flexibility, balance, and overall well-being.

<u>Here are some important basic practices:</u>

- ❖ **Seated Breathing Exercises:**
  - ➢ Sit comfortably in a firm chair, feet flat on the ground.
  - ➢ Close your eyes and take a few slow, profound breaths. Inhale through your nose, extend your chest and abdomen, then exhale through your mouth.
  - ➢ Concentrate on the present moment, letting go of any worry and tension.
- ❖ **Gentle Neck Stretches:**
  - ➢ Sit upright in your chair.
  - ➢ Gently tilt your head to the right, placing your right ear near your right shoulder. Hold for a few breaths.
  - ➢ Repeat on the left side.
  - ➢ This helps to relieve tension in the neck and shoulders.
- ❖ **Shoulder Rolls:**
  - ➢ Move your shoulders forward in a circular motion, then reverse.
  - ➢ This reduces stiffness and improves circulation.
- ❖ Perform a seated Cat-Cow stretch by placing your hands on your thighs.
  - ➢ Inhale, arch your back, and raise your chest (cow stance).

- ➢ Exhale, round your back, and tuck your chin (cat stance).
- ➢ Repeat multiple repetitions, synchronizing movement and breath.
- ❖ **Ankle Circles:** Lift one foot off the ground and rotate your ankle clockwise and counterclockwise.
  - ➢ Switch to the other foot.
  - ➢ Ankle circles increase circulation and ankle flexibility.
- ❖ **Seated Forward Fold:**
  - ➢ Sit on the edge of your chair.
  - ➢ Inhale, lengthen your spine, and extend your arms forwards.
  - ➢ Exhale, hinge at the hips, and fold gently forward.
  - ➢ Feel a Lengthen in your hamstrings and lower back.
- ❖ **Mindful Relaxation:**
  - ➢ Close your eyes and concentrate on breathing.
  - ➢ Visualize a warm, relaxing glow flowing throughout your body.
  - ➢ Let rid of any tension and allow your muscles to fully relax.

Remember, chair yoga is all about respecting your body's limitations and tailoring practices to your comfort level. Always listen to your body, and if something doesn't feel right, adjust or skip it.

Regular practice can help you become more flexible, reduce stress, and feel better overall. Feel free to try out these techniques and gradually incorporate them into your everyday routine.

Basic Poses and Movements

Let's look at some basic chair yoga postures and motions that are ideal for seniors over 60. These simple exercises can be done seated to improve flexibility, balance, and overall well-being.

- ❖ **Seated Mountain Pose (Tadasana)**
  - ➢ Sit tall in your chair, feet flat on the ground.
  - ➢ Put your hands on your thighs or knees.
  - ➢ Extend your spine, raise your chest, and relax your shoulders.
  - ➢ Take deep breaths and feel anchored.
- ❖ **Chair Cat-Cow Stretch:**
  - ➢ Sit on the edge of your chair.
  - ➢ Inhale, arch your back, and raise your chest (cow stance).
  - ➢ Exhale, round your back, and tuck your chin (cat stance).
  - ➢ Repeat the gentle spinal movement many times.
- ❖ **Seated Forward Bend (Paschimottanasana)**
  - ➢ Sit at the front of your chair.
  - ➢ Inhale, lengthen your spine, and extend your arms forwards.
  - ➢ Exhale, hinge at the hips, and fold gently forward.
  - ➢ Feel a Lengthen in your hamstrings and low back.
- ❖ **Seated Twist (Ardha Matsyendrasana):**
  - ➢ Sit sideways in your chair.
  - ➢ With one hand, hold the backrest while the other rests on the opposite thigh.
  - ➢ Inhale, extend your spine, and gently twist to the side.
  - ➢ Exhale and deepen the twist.
  - ➢ Switch sides and repeat.

- ❖ **Ankle Circles:** Lift one foot off the ground and rotate your ankle clockwise and counterclockwise.
  - ➤ Switch to the other foot.
  - ➤ Ankle circles increase circulation and ankle flexibility.
- ❖ **Seated Leg Lifts:**
  - ➤ Sit tall and stretch one straight leg.
  - ➤ Flex your foot and raise your leg a few inches from the ground.
  - ➤ Lower it back down.
  - ➤ Repeat with the opposite leg.
  - ➤ This strengthens the quadriceps and boosts leg circulation.
- ❖ **Seated Shoulder Opener.**
  - ➤ Position your hands behind your back.
  - ➤ Straighten and lift your arms slightly.
  - ➤ Extend your chest and softly raise your chin.
  - ➤ Release and repeat as necessary.

Muse on that chair yoga is about adjusting poses to your comfort level. Listen to your body, breathe deliberately, and reap the benefits of this simple practice.

Creating a Routine: The 28-day Beginner Challenge

Starting a chair yoga journey may be thrilling and transformative. Whether you're a senior over 60 or seeking for a light practice, a well-structured program can make a big difference. In this 28-day beginner challenge, we'll walk you through a gentle progression to help you develop strength, flexibility, and awareness. Remember that consistency is essential, and each day's practice improves your general well-being.

Week 1: Foundation and Breathing Awareness

- ❖ **Day One:** Seated Breathing Awareness
  - ➢ Take a comfortable seat in your chair.
  - ➢ -Shut your eyes and concentrate on your respiration.
  - ➢ Take deep breaths through your nose, stretching your chest and abdomen.
  - ➢ Slowly exhale through your mouth.
  - ➢ Practice for five minutes.
- • **Day 7:** Gentle Neck Stretches
  - ➢ Sit tall with your head softly tilted to the right.
  - ➢ Pause for a few breaths before switching sides.
  - ➢ Reduce stiffness in your neck and shoulders.

Week Two: Mobility and Balance

- ❖ **Day 14:** Seated Cat-Cow Stretch
  - ➢ Alternate between arched back (cow pose) and rounded spine (cat pose).
  - ➢ Coordinate movement with breath.
  - ➢ Repeat ten times.
- ❖ **Day 21,** Ankle Circles and Leg Lifts
  - ➢ Raise one foot from the ground and rotate your ankle.
  - ➢ Switch to the other foot.
  - ➢ Next, elevate each leg to strengthen your quadriceps.

Week Three: Strength and Flexibility

- ❖ **Day 15:** Seated Forward Bend
  - ➢ Sit on the edge of your chair.

> Inhale, lengthen your spine, and extend your arms forwards.

> Exhale, hinge at the hips, and fold gently forward.

> Feel a stretch in your hamstrings.

❖ **Day 22:** Seated Twist.

> Sit sideways in your chair.

> Twist gently to the side while clutching the backrest.

> Take a deep breath and remove any stress.

Week Four: Mindfulness and Relaxation

❖ **Day 28:** Mindful Relaxation.

> Strong matches your eyes and focus on your breathing.

> Imagine warmth spreading throughout your body.

> Release of the stress and strain.

> Practice for ten minutes.

- **Tip for Success:**

  > **Consistency:** Set aside time every day to practice, even if it's only for a few minutes.

  > **Modify positions:** Adjust positions to suit your comfort level. Listen to your body.

  > **Props:** Consider using a pillow or folded blanket for support.

  > **Enjoy the Journey:** Recognize minor wins and relish the experience.

Look back on that chair yoga is more than just physical movement; it is about linking the mind, body, and breath. As you finish this 28-day challenge, you will gain new strength, balance, and inner calm. Please check your healthcare physician before beginning any new workout regimen, especially if you have certain health conditions.

Modifications and Adaptations for Beginners

Let's look at some crucial modifications and adaptations for chair yoga novices. These modifications enable a safe and successful practice, especially for senior citizens over 60 or those new to yoga.

- ❖ Select and place a sturdy, armless chair with a flat seat. Avoid chairs with wheels.
  - ➢ **Positioning:** Place the chair on a non-slip surface so it does not move during practice.
- ❖ **Mindful Approach:**
  - ➢ **Listen to your body:** Pay attention to how your body feels while in each stance. Discomfort or pain is a warning to change.
  - ➢ Breathe: Concentrate on calm, deep breaths. Breathing promotes calm and keeps you present.
- ❖ **Seated Poses:**
  - ➢ **Seat Height:** Adjust chair height as appropriate. "Ensure that your feet are flat on the ground."

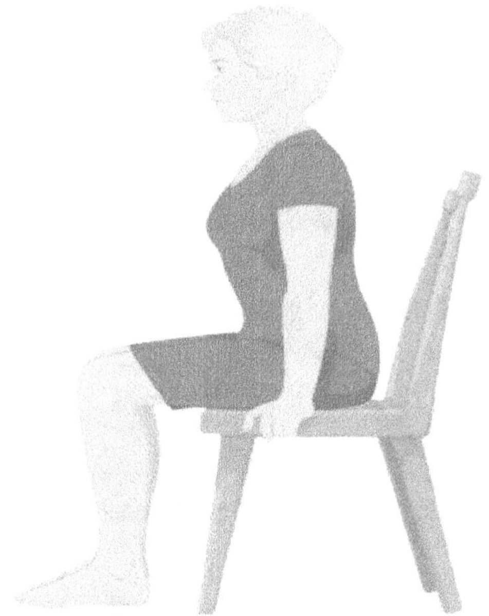

➢ **Spinal Alignment:** Sit tall to stretch your spine. Imagine a cord tugging you up.

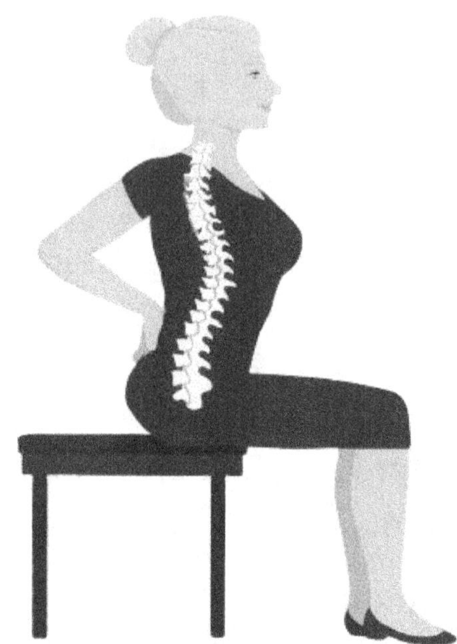

➢ **Supported backbends:** Use the backrest to perform mild backbends. Avoid excessive arching.

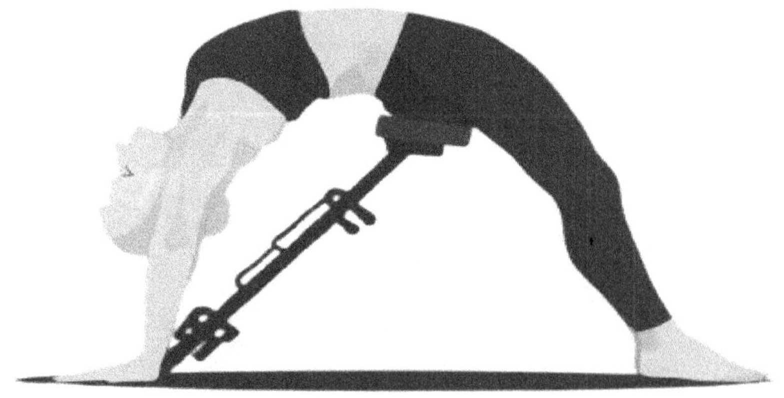

- ❖ **Joint-Friendly Movements:**
  - ➢ **Gentle Range of Motion:** Move joints smoothly and without force. Avoid quick or jerky movements.
  - ➢ **Circles for the ankle and wrist:** Warm up your ankles and wrists by rotating them in both directions.
- ❖ **Breathing Techniques:**
  - ➢ Diaphragmatic Breathing Practice deep belly breathing. Inhale as your abdomen expands and exhale when it contracts.
  - ➢ **Counted breaths:** Inhale for four counts, then exhale for six. Gradually extend your exhalation.
- ❖ **Adapted Poses:**
  - ➢ **Seated Mountain Pose:** Sit tall with hands on thighs. Inhale, lengthening the spine; exhale, relaxing the shoulders.

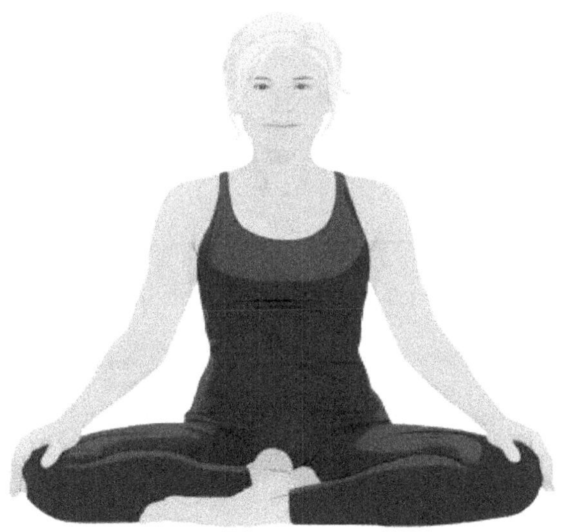

➢ **Seated Forward Fold:** Hinge at the hips and stretch forward. Modify by slightly bending the knees.

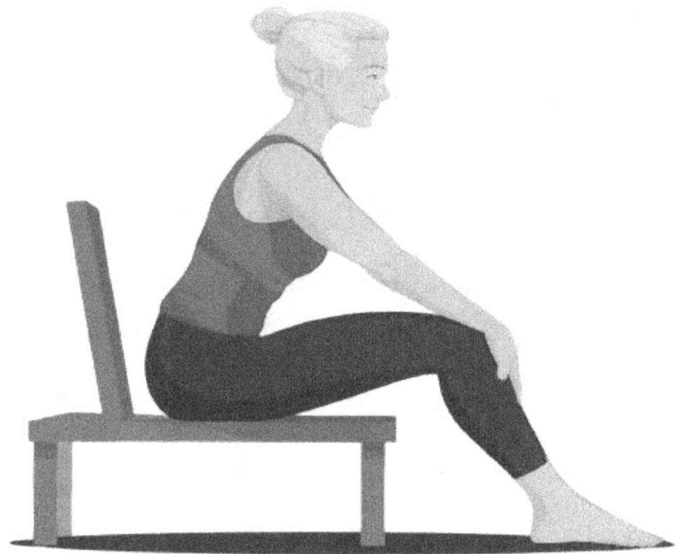

➢ **The Seated Twist:** Twist gently, using the chair's backrest as support.

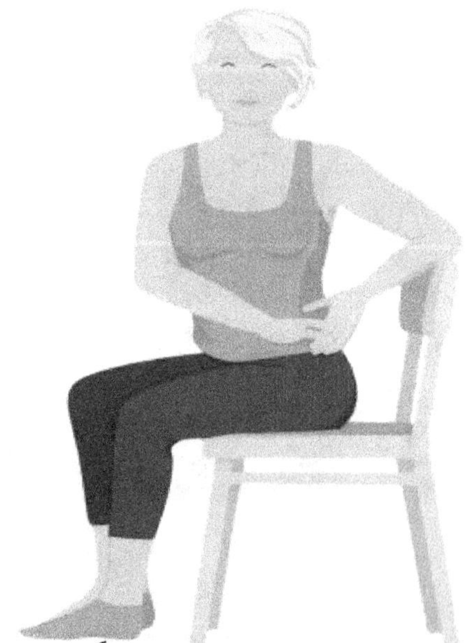

- ❖ **Props and Support:**
  - ➢ **Blankets or Cushions:** Place under hips for extra comfort.
  - ➢ **Strap or Belt:** Use to stretch if reaching your feet is difficult.
  - ➢ **Wall Support:** Sit near a wall for stability when performing balance poses.
- ❖ **Mindset and Patience:**
  - ➢ **Non-judgment:** Let go of expectations. Every practice represents growth.
  - ➢ **Patience:** Give yourself time to learn and adjust. Rome wasn't constructed in one day!
- ❖ **Common Conditions and Modifications:**
  - ➢ **Arthritis:** Use gentle movements and avoid tight grips.
  - ➢ **Osteoporosis:** Avoid doing deep forward bends or twists.
  - ➢ If you have hip or knee problems, modify your leg lifts and seated positions.
  - ➢ **Balance Concerns:** Use the chair as a support during balance workouts.
- ❖ **Warm-Up and Cool-Down:**
  - ➢ Begin with neck stretches, shoulder rolls, and ankle circles.
  - ➢ **Cool-Down:** Finish with a seated relaxation while focusing on your breath.

Remember that chair yoga is about meeting your body's demands. Adaptations allow you to enjoy your practice while avoiding strain. Before beginning any new workout regimen, see your healthcare professional, especially if you have any specific health concerns. Enjoy your chair yoga trip! Please keep in mind that this information is provided solely for educational reasons and is not intended to replace professional advice.

Chapter 7: Intermediate Chair Yoga Practices

Intermediate chair yoga practices expand on the core exercises, providing deeper stretches, increased strength, and improved mindfulness. Let's look at some crucial aspects of an intermediate chair yoga practice:

- ❖ **Standing with Chair Support:**
  - ➢ **Warrior Poses:** Adapted variations of Warrior I and Warrior II can be practiced using the chair for balance. These positions work the thighs, hips, and core.
  - ➢ **Tree pose:** Stand near the chair and place one foot on the inner thigh of the opposing leg. The chair gives support as you learn to balance.
- ❖ **Twists and Spinal Mobility:**
  - ➢ **Seated Twists:** Practice mild twists while sitting. Hold the backrest and twist from the waist, allowing the spine to stretch.
  - ➢ **Chair Revolved Triangle:** A seated twist in which one leg extends forward and the other foot is positioned against the chair. Twist towards the extended leg.
- ❖ **Backbends and Heart Openers:**
  - ➢ **Seated Backbends:** Arch backward using the chair's support to stretch the front body and open the chest.
  - ➢ **Supported Camel Pose:** Kneel in front of the chair with your hands on the seat and gently arch backward.
- ❖ **Balance Challenges:**

- **Single-Leg Balance:** Stand on one leg while elevating the other foot off the ground. Hold on to the chair for stability.
- **Chair Eagle Pose.** Cross one leg over the other and wrap the foot around the calf. Extend your arms like eagle wings.
- ❖ **Mindfulness and Breath Awareness:**
- **Ujjayi Breathing:** Take deep, ocean-like breaths. Inhale via the nose and exhale audibly through the mouth.
- **Mindful transitions:** Pay attention to how you transition from one stance to another. Maintain awareness of your body and breathing.
- ❖ **Strength-Building Variations:**
- **Chair Plank:**
  - ➢ Place hands on chair seat, step back into plank posture, and engage core.
- **Chair Chaturanga:** Lower your elbows halfway down, keeping them close to your body.
- ❖ **Use Props:**
  - ➢ Use a strap or belt for shoulder stretches or deepening forward folds.
- **Blanket or Cushion:** Provides support for the knees and hips while seate
- ❖ **Mind-Body Connection:**
  - ➢ **Visualization:** Imagine energy flowing through your body while holding each stance.
  - ➢ **Affirmations:** Use positive remarks discreetly to improve your practice.

Remember, consistency and patience are essential. As you develop, acknowledge your body's limitations and applaud minor accomplishments. Consult your healthcare professional before beginning any new fitness regimen, especially if you have specific health conditions.

Intermediate Poses for Enhanced Mobility and Strength

Intermediate yoga poses serve as a transition between foundational and advanced postures. They offer an exciting opportunity to improve core strength, balance, flexibility, and overall mobility.

<u>Let's look at several crucial intermediate positions that can improve your practice:</u>

- ❖ **Benefits of Dancer Pose II (Natarajasana II)** include improved balance and   focus.
  - ➢ Stretches the quadriceps, hip flexors, and shoulders.
  - ➢ It strengthens the standing leg and core.
- **How to Practice:**
  - ➢ Stand tall and move your weight to one leg.
  - ➢ Bend the opposing knee and reach back to support the foot or ankle.
  - ➢ Extend your other arm forward.
  - ➢ Maintain a steady gaze and take deep breaths
- ❖ **Benefits of Archer Pose (Akarna Dhanurasana):**
  - ➢ Opens the chest and shoulders.
  - ➢ Strengthens the legs and increases hip flexibility.
- **How to Practice:**
  - ➢ Stand with your feet apart.
  - ➢ Extend one foot and bend your knee.
  - ➢ Reach the same-side arm forward and the opposite arm back.
  - ➢ Imagine drawing a bowstring.

- ❖ **Benefits of Standing Wind Relieving Pose (Utthita Vayu Muktasana)**
  - ➢ Stimulates the digestive system.
  - ➢ Stretches the hips and hamstrings.
- **How to Practice:**
  - ➢ Stand with your feet hip width apart.
  - ➢ Raise one knee to the chest.
  - ➢ Hold onto the knee with both hands.
  - ➢ Take deep breaths and maintain equilibrium.
- ❖ **Twist Half Chair Pose (Parivrtta Ardha Utkatasana):**
- **Benefits:**
  - ➢ Strengthens legs and core.
  - ➢ Promotes spinal mobility.
- ❖ **How to Practice:**
  - ➢ Start in a half-chair pose (squat position).
  - ➢ Twist your torso to one side, bringing the opposing elbow outside the knee.
  - ➢ Keep your spine long and breathe through the twist.
- ❖ **Bound Half Moon Twist (Baddha Parivrtta Half Moon):**
- ❖ **Benefits:**
  - ➢ Requires balance and coordination.
  - ➢ Improves hip and hamstring mobility.
- ❖ **How to Practice:**
  - ➢ From Half Moon Pose, bend your elevated knee.
  - ➢ Reach back with the same-side hand to grab the foot.
  - ➢ Balance on one leg and gently twist your torso.

- ❖ **Benefits of Standing Forward Bend (Ardha Baddha Padmottanasana):**
  - ➤ Stretches hamstrings and calves.
  - ➤ Improves balance and concentration.
- ❖ **How to Practice:**
  - ➤ Stand tall, lift one leg, and place foot on inner thigh.
  - ➤ Fold forward and grasp for the ground or ankle.
  - ➤ Extend the spine and breathe deeply.
- ❖ **Benefits of Upward Facing Wide-Angle Seated Pose (Urdhva Upavistha Konasana)** include opening the inner thighs and groin.
  - ➤ Sure, here is the revised text:
  - ➤ "It helps to strengthen the core and back."
- ❖ **Practice:**
  - ➤ Sit with legs wide apart.
  - ➤ Extend the spine and fold forward.
  - ➤ Extend the arms or grip the feet.
- ❖ **Reclined Intense Back Stretch Pose (Supta Paschimottanasana):**
- ❖ **Benefits:**
  - ➤ Relaxes spine and hamstrings.
  - ➤ Relaxes the nervous system.
- • **How to Practice:**
  - ➤ Lie on your back.
  - ➤ Extend the legs upward and flex the feet.
  - ➤ Reach for the toes or ankles.

Not lose sight of the fact that consistency and patience are crucial. Always listen to your body, make adjustments as needed, and grow at your own pace. These intermediate poses will improve your practice and promote your general well-being.

Creating a Routine: The 28-day Intermediate Challenge

Let's start by constructing a 28-day intermediate challenge routine that includes strength, flexibility, and mindfulness. Whether you're starting from scratch or increasing your practice, this strategy will help you make good progress. Consult your healthcare professional before beginning any new fitness regimen, especially if you have specific health conditions.

Developing a Routine: The 28-Day Intermediate Challenge

Week One: Foundation and Strength

- ❖ **Day One: Dynamic Warm-up**
  - ➢ Begin with 5 minutes of easy cardio (jumping jacks and high knees).
  - ➢ Do bodyweight squats, lunges, and push-ups.
  - ➢ Concentrate on form and activation.
- ❖ **Day 7: Upper Body Strength.**
  - ➢ Push-ups: three sets of 10 to 12 reps.
  - ➢ Dips (with a sturdy chair): three sets of ten reps.
  - ➢ Plank: Hold for 30-60 seconds.

Week Two: Flexibility and Balance

- ❖ **Day 14: Yoga Flow.**
  - ➢ **Sun Salutations:** Practice downward dog, plank, cobra, and upward dog.

- ➤ **Warrior Pose:** Strengthen legs and open hips.
- ❖ **Day 21 Balance Challenge**
  - ➤ **Tree Pose:** Stand on one leg with hands at the heart center.
  - ➤ **Single-Leg Deadlifts:** Hinge forward and extend one leg behind you.

Week Three: Core and Mindfulness

- ❖ **Day 15: Core Circuit**
  - ➤ Bicycle Crunches (3 sets of 20 reps).
  - ➤ **Russian Twists:** three sets of 12 reps.
- ❖ **Day 22: Mindful Meditation.**
  - ➤ Sit comfortable and close your eyes.
  - ➤ For ten minutes, pay attention to your breathing.
  - ➤ Be at peace with the arising and going of thoughts.

Week 4: Full Body Challenge

- ❖ **Day 28: HIIT Workout.**
  - ➤ High Intensity Interval Training (HIIT):
  - ➤ Jump squats for 30 seconds
  - ➤ Mountain climbers: thirty seconds.
  - ➤ Rest for 30 seconds.
  - ➤ Repeat for three rounds.
- • **Tip for Success:**
  - ➤ **Progressive Overload:** Gradually increase your reps, sets, or intensity.
  - ➤ **Listen to Your Body:** Modify as needed to avoid overtraining.
  - ➤ **Rest and Recovery:** Schedule at least one rest day every week.
  - ➤ **Hydrate and Fuel:** Stay hydrated and eat nutritious meals.
  - ➤ **Celebrate Milestones:** Recognize your progress!

Remember that consistency is crucial. Enjoy the task, stay inspired, and celebrate your accomplishments. Please check your healthcare provider before beginning any new exercise program.

Advancing Your Practice Safely

Let's go more into *"Advancing Your Practice Safely"* in the context of chair yoga for elders.

- ❖ **Progress Gradually:**
  - ➤ Once you're comfortable with fundamental chair yoga positions, gradually add variations or deeper stretches. For example:
- ❖ **Modified Twists:** Begin with gentle seated twists that engage the core and spine. As you develop, try deeper rotations.
- ❖ **Extended Arm Stretches:** Start with easy arm lifts while sitting. Gradually extend your arms higher or try diagonal stretches.
- ❖ **Leg Extensions:** Initially, lift your legs slightly off the ground to strengthen. As you progress, aim for higher leg lifts or ankle circles.
- ❖ **Remember:** safety comes first. If any movement is uncomfortable or painful, alter or avoid it.
- ❖ **Mindful Breathing Techniques:**
  - ➤ Deep, aware breathing improves your practice. Focus on diaphragmatic breathing, which involves breathing deeply into your gut and stretching your ribcage. This relaxes the nervous system and increases lung capacity.
- ❖ **Counted breaths:** Inhale for four counts, hold for two, and then exhale for six. To suit your comfort level, Ajust the counts.

- **Ocean Breath (Ujjayi):** Make a quiet ocean-like sound by restricting your throat during inhale and exhale. It promotes both relaxation and concentration.

  - ❖ **Balance Challenges:**
    - ➢ Practice balance-enhancing positions while sitting.
  - ❖ **Single-Leg Lifts:** Lift one foot off the ground while activating your core. Gradually extend the duration and repetitions.

- **Heel-Toe Taps:** Tap your heels or toes alternatively to maintain stability. Close your eyes briefly to challenge yourself.

  - ❖ **Side Reach:** Raise one arm overhead while elevating the opposing leg. Switch sides for balance and coordination.
  - ❖ **Mindfulness and Focus:**
    - ➢ Chair yoga is more than simply physical movement; it also involves mindfulness. Pay attention to:
  - ❖ **Body Awareness:** Be aware of sensations, alignment, and muscular engagement.
  - ❖ **Thoughts and Emotion:** Observe without passing judgment. If your thoughts wander, gently draw them back to the present moment.
  - ❖ **Gratitude:** Be grateful for your body's abilities and the chance to practice. seated meditation for a few minutes at the end of your practice. Close your eyes, concentrate on your breath, and let your thoughts come and go.
    - ➢ Use a simple mantra, such as ***"I am calm,"*** to help you focus.

Call to mind that improving your practice does not imply pushing yourself to extremes. It is about progressive development, self-awareness, and respecting your body's demands. Enjoy your adventure!

Chapter 8: Advanced Chair Yoga Practices

Advanced chair yoga techniques allow seniors over 60 to improve their well-being, flexibility, and strength.

Let's get onto the main points:

- ❖ **Seated Eagle Pose:** Cross one leg over the other, entwining your arms. It tests balance and coordination while increasing stability.
- ❖ **Chair Warrior Pose:** Adapted from the conventional Warrior Pose, this variation works the legs, arms, and core. It assists seniors to stay strong and functional.
- ❖ **Breathing Techniques and Relaxation:** Chair yoga focuses on attentive breathing and guided meditations. These routines relieve stress, improve mental clarity, and promote general health.
- ❖ **Flexibility Poses:** Work on upper and lower body flexibility. These mild exercises promote mobility and alleviate stiffness.
- ❖ **Strength-Building Poses:** Work on the core, arms, and legs. Chair yoga is an excellent workout for preserving physical wellness.
- ❖ **Balance and Stability:** Practice specialized workouts to improve your balance. Improved balance lowers the chance of falling and increases confidence.
- ❖ **Community Connection:** Chair yoga promotes a sense of community by offering elders support and encouragement.

Always remember, consistency is important! Daily chair yoga can provide considerable health benefits. For more extensive advice, consider studying resources like the book "Chair Yoga for seniors over 60".

Advanced Poses for Deepening Flexibility and Stamina

Advanced yoga postures are complex and physically demanding, requiring extraordinary strength, flexibility, balance, and body awareness. These poses go beyond the basics, frequently include deep stretches, intricate transitions, and variations.

Let's look at some advanced positions that help increase flexibility and stamina:

- ❖ **Handstand Split:** This posture involves kicking up into a handstand and then splitting your legs apart to form an elegant V shape. It tests your core, shoulders, and hip flexibility.

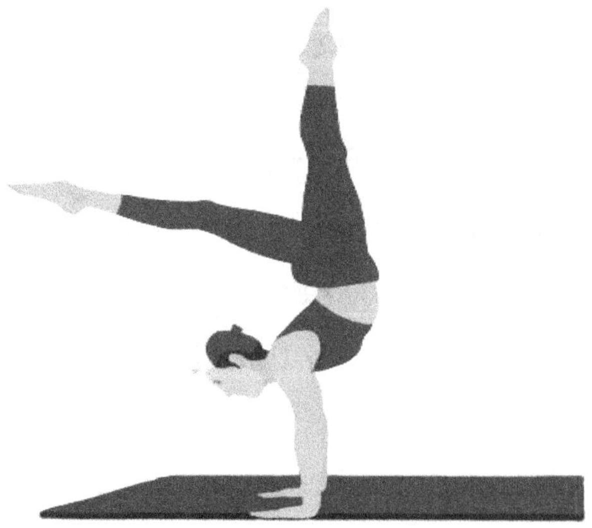

❖ **One-Arm Handstand:** The one-arm handstand is the pinnacle of strength and balance, requiring you to support your entire body weight with one arm while remaining stable. It necessitates significant core involvement and shoulder strength

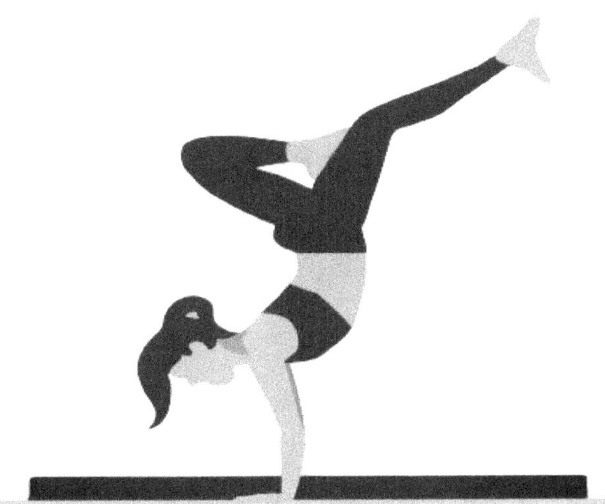

❖ **Mexican Handstand:** The Mexican handstand is similar to a forearm stand in that you balance on your forearms with your legs extended upward. It's a great approach to improve shoulder flexibility and upper-body strength.

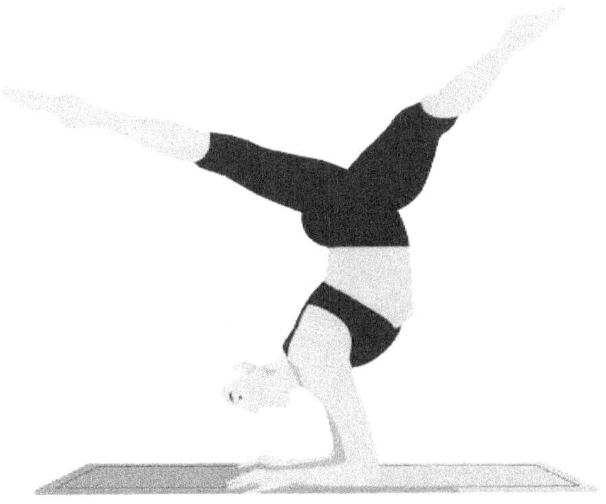

❖ **Hollowback Handstand:** This variant involves arching your back while in a handstand, resulting in a gorgeous curve. It requires both strength and spinal flexibility.

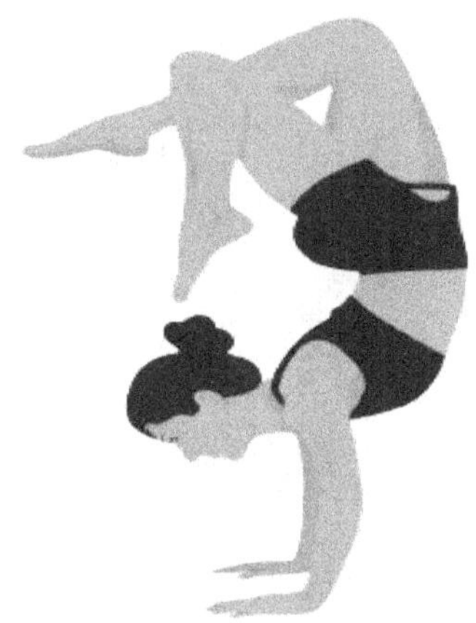

❖ **Tuck Handstand:** In this handstand variation, your legs are tucked near your chest rather than fully extended. It's a step toward more sophisticated handstands.

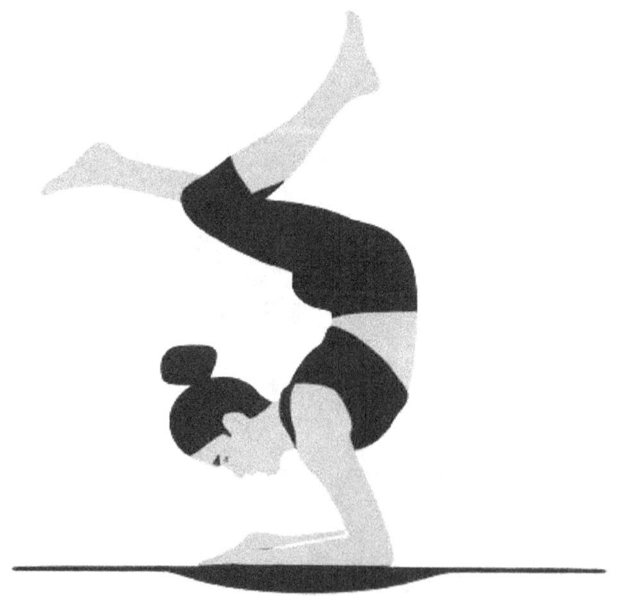

❖ **Straddle Handstand:** You extend your legs wide apart while upside down. It tests hip flexibility and balance.

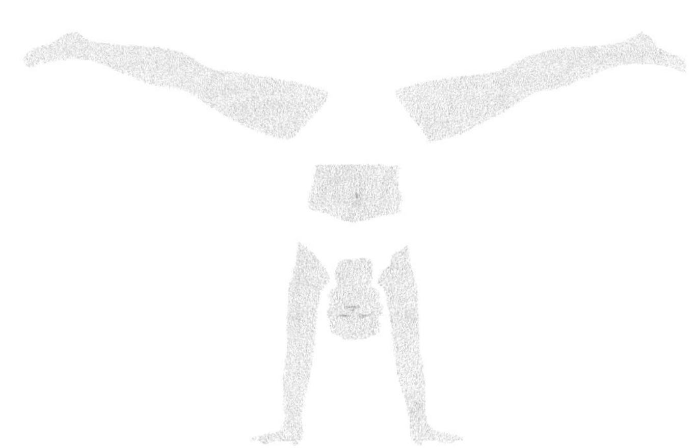

❖ **Press Handstand:** This pose requires raising into a handstand without jumping. It necessitates extreme core strength and control. Take into consideration that advanced poses require patience, perseverance, and adequate supervision.

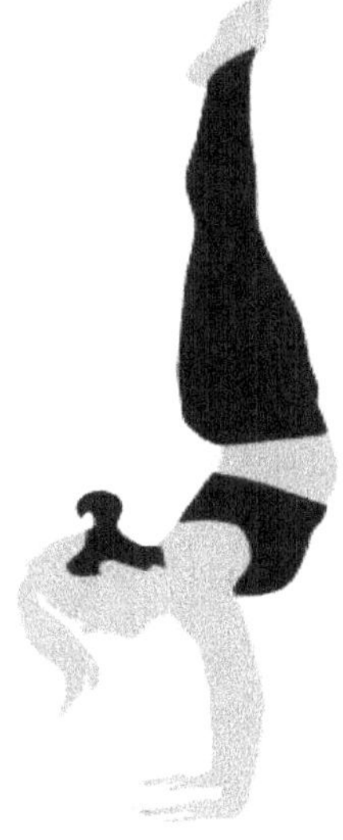

NEVER forget to listen to your body and warm up properly. These poses not only improve physical ability but also strengthen the mind-body connection and spiritual awareness.

Creating a Routine: The 28-day Advanced Challenge

Let's dive into the **28-Day Advanced Challenge,** a transforming practice that will improve your strength, flexibility, and stamina. This challenge goes beyond the basics, testing your limits and encouraging improvement.

<u>Below is how to develop a successful 28-day routine:</u>

- ❖ **Goal Setting and Commitment:** Clarify your objectives. Are you looking to improve flexibility, muscle endurance, or both?
  - ➤ Fully commit to the challenge. Consistency is essential.
- ❖ **Structured Workouts:**
  - ➤ Break down the challenge into four seven-day segments.
  - ➤ Concentrate on certain body parts: upper body, lower body, core, and full-body workouts.
  - ➤ Incorporate advanced postures such as handstands, splits, and hollow backs.
- ❖ **Warm-Up and Cool-Down:**
  - ➤ Start each session with dynamic stretches to prepare your muscles.
  - ➤ Finish with static stretches to increase flexibility and avoid injury.

- ❖ **Progressive Overload:** gradually increase intensity. Increase the number of reps, hold positions for longer, or change exercises.
  - ➢ Track your progress to keep yourself motivated.
- ❖ **Nutrition and Hydration:**
  - ➢ Consume balanced meals high in protein, healthy fats, and carbohydrates.
  - ➢ Stay hydrated during the challenge.
- ❖ **Rest and Recovery:**
  - ➢ Allow for muscle repair and growth.
  - ➢ Include rest days or active rehabilitation activities (for example, gentle yoga or walking).
- ❖ **Mind-Body Connection:** Yoga is not only physical, but also mental.
  - ➢ Practice mindfulness throughout your sessions. Take deep breaths and stay present. Not forget that the 28-day advanced challenge is primarily about making progress, not perfectionism. Listen to your body, make adjustments as needed, and celebrate tiny triumphs along the road.

Mastering Chair Yoga Techniques

Let look into the art of **Mastering Chair Yoga Techniques,** which is specifically designed for seniors over 60. Chair yoga combines moderate movements, breath awareness, and mindfulness, all while sitting. It improves flexibility, balance, and overall well-being. Below are the main points to master:

- ❖ **Seated Mountain Pose (Tadasana):**
  - ➢ Sit tall in your chair, feet flat on the ground.
  - ➢ Keep your spine aligned, your shoulders relaxed, and your core engaged.
  - ➢ Take deep breaths and feel anchored.

- ❖ **Seated Forward Fold (Paschimottanasana):** Sit on the edge of your chair.
  - ➢ Hinge at the hips and extend forward with a straight spine.
  - ➢ You should feel a stretch in your hamstrings and low back.
- ❖ **Seated Twist (Ardha Matsyendrasana):** Sit sideways in your chair.
  - ➢ Hold the backrest with one hand and gradually twist your torso.
  - ➢ This posture increases spinal mobility and facilitates digestion.
- ❖ **Seated Cat-Cow Stretch:** Place hands on thighs.
  - ➢ Inhale, arch your back (cow stance), and raise your chest.
  - ➢ Exhale, circle your spine (cat position), and tuck your chin.
  - ➢ Repeat for a moderate spinal warmup.
- ❖ **Ankle-to-Knee Stretch:** Bring your right ankle over the left knee.
  - ➢ Gently press down on your right knee to experience a hip stretch.
  - ➢ Switch sides.
- ❖ **Seated Warrior (Virabhadrasana):** Extend one leg forward while bending the other knee.
  - ➢ Raise your arms upward with palms facing each other.
  - ➢ Engage your core and take deep breaths.
- ❖ **Chair Pigeon Pose:** Cross your right ankle over your left thigh.
  - ➢ Flex your right foot and slowly lean forward.
  - ➢ Feel a stretch in your hips and gluteS.
- ❖ **Breathing Awareness:**
  - ➢ Practice deep and attentive breathing.
  - ➢ Inhale through your nostrils and stretch your ribcage.
  - ➢ Exhale slowly to relieve stress.
- ❖ **Neck and Shoulder Relaxation:**
  - ➢ Lower your right ear to your right shoulder.

- ➤ Gently stretch your neck.
- ➤ Switch sides.
- ❖ **Mindfulness Meditation:** Close your eyes and concentrate on your breathing.
  - ➤ Avoid distractions and focus on the present moment.

Keep in mind, chair yoga is about respecting your body's limitations. Pay attention to your body and modify the poses as needed. Consistency and patience will result in progress.

Chapter 9: Specialized Chair Yoga Programs

<u>Let's look into specific chair yoga programs, focusing on what makes them unique:</u>

- ❖ **Adaptive and Inclusive Workouts:**
  - ➢ These programs cater to a wide range of requirements, including seniors, people with impairments, and those recovering from injuries.
  - ➢ Instructors modify poses and sequences to meet physical restrictions, allowing everyone to participate.
  - ➢ The emphasis is on accessibility, making yoga an inclusive practice for everybody.
- ❖ **Mindful Breathing Techniques:**
  - ➢ Specialized chair yoga emphasizes breath awareness.
  - ➢ Participants are taught techniques like as **"Ujjayi"** (victorious breath) to soothe the mind and promote relaxation.
  - ➢ Concentrating on the breath promotes awareness, reduces stress, and increases mental clarity.
- ❖ **Seated Meditation and Visualization:**
  - ➢ Chair yoga classes typically involve guided meditation while sitting.
  - ➢ Participants envision healing energy, positivity, or specific aspirations.
  - ➢ This exercise promotes emotional well-being and inner tranquility.
- ❖ **Chair-Based Strength Building:**
  - ➢ Unique exercises target specific muscle areas utilizing a chair as a prop.
  - ➢ Examples are "Seated Warrior" (for upper body strength) and "Chair Squats" (for lower body strength).

Seniors benefit from increased muscle tone and functional strength.

- ❖ **Joint Mobility and Flexibility:**
  - ➤ Specialized programs promote mild joint movements.
  - ➤ Participants investigate circular motions for the wrists, ankles, and shoulders.
  - ➤ These motions improve joint health and reduce stiffness.
- ❖ **Chair Yoga for Chronic concerns:**
  - ➤ Some programs focus on specific health concerns.
  - ➤ For example, **"Arthritis Chair Yoga"** focuses on joint-friendly positions.
  - ➤ Participants get alleviation from pain and inflammation.
- ❖ **Social Connection and Community:**
  - ➤ Chair yoga courses promote a sense of belonging.
  - ➤ Seniors interact with others, share their experiences, and form connections.
  - ➤ The supportive environment promotes general well-being. Take into account that specialized chair yoga programs focus on specific needs, making them an invaluable resource for seniors seeking holistic wellness.
  - ➤

Chair Yoga for Senior's

Chair yoga is a mild yoga practice that aims to improve the well-being, flexibility, and mental health of seniors over the age of 60. It entails adapting conventional postures to seated positions or using a chair for support. Chair yoga provides increased flexibility, strength, posture, stress reduction, and energy flow. The basic chair yoga positions include sitting mountain pose, sitting forward fold, sitting twist, sitting cat-cow, and sitting warrior. Mindful breathing, using props to modify poses, and staying consistent are all good practice techniques. Chair yoga emphasizes gentle movement, self-awareness, and respect for the body. You are encouraged to share this practice with other elders and enjoy the experience.

Chair Yoga for Office Workers

Chair yoga for office workers is an effective way to improve physical health, mental well-being, and productivity.

<u>Some factors to consider:</u>

- ❖ **Structure Your Day:** Set aside distinct blocks of time for chair yoga in the morning and afternoon. Even brief sessions can make an impact.
- ❖ **Pose Wisely:** Not all positions are appropriate for an office atmosphere. Choose mild stretches that will not impede your workflow. Examples include neck rolls, seated forward folds, and shoulder stretches.
- ❖ **Mindful Movement:** Before you begin, check in with your body. Pay attention to any tenseness or pain. Move with mindfulness, focusing on alignment and breath awareness.
- ❖ **Breath Awareness:** Add aware breathing to your practice. Deep, regular breathing can help relieve tension and improve focus.
- ❖ **Use Props:** Use office supplies such as a strong chair or desk for support. Props provide stability and allow for deeper stretches.

Remember that chair yoga provides more than simply physical advantages; it also serves as a mental reset. Integrating these techniques into your workday will improve your general well-being while still maintaining productivity.

Chair Yoga for Rehabilitation and Physical Therapy

Chair yoga is a gentle exercise that combines physical movement, mindfulness, and relaxation. It is particularly beneficial for rehabilitation and physical therapy, especially for seniors and those with limited mobility. Chair yoga improves joint flexibility, strength, balance, posture, and mental and emotional well-being. It aids in injury recovery, chronic conditions, and stroke recovery. Adapted poses include sitting forward fold, sitting twist, ankle circles, and breathing exercises. It is important to consult a healthcare provider, listen to your body, and maintain consistency in practice.

Chapter 10: Integrating Chair Yoga into Daily Life

Integrating chair yoga into your daily routine has numerous advantages, whether you're a busy professional, a senior, or recovering from an injury.

<u>Let's look at how you can smoothly include this easy technique into your routine:</u>

- ❖ **Morning Wake-Up Routine:** Start the day with a few minutes of chair yoga. Sit upright in your chair, close your eyes, and take deep breaths. Gently extend your arms upwards, twist your torso, and awaken your spine. This creates a pleasant tone for the day.
- ❖ **Desk Breaks:** If you work in a sedentary environment, try chair yoga as a lunchtime recharge. Stretch the neck, shoulders, and wrists. Try seated cat-cow stretches to relieve tension. To refresh your mind, concentrate on your breathing.
- ❖ **Lunchtime Practice:**
  - ➢ **Find a quiet area during lunchtime:** Practice seated forward folds, ankle circles, and wrist rotations. These movements aid digestion and prevent stiffness.
- ❖ **Afternoon Energy Boost:**
  - ➢ Feeling sluggish? Try seated sun salutations. Inhale, raise your arms, then exhale and fold them forward. Energize your body without leaving your seat.

- ❖ **Evening Relaxation:** Relax with gentle twists. Sit sideways in your chair, holding the backrest and twisting your upper body. Inhale deeply. This relieves tension and gets you ready for a good night's sleep.
- ❖ **TV Time or Reading:** Combine leisure and enjoyment. While watching television or reading, perform ankle pumps, sitting leg lifts, or shoulder rolls. Multitasking is effortless.
- ❖ **When waiting in lines or commuting, practice chair yoga during downtime.** While you wait, keep yourself grounded with ankle rotations, seated spinal twists, and deep breaths.
- ❖ **before Bed Ritual:**
  - ➤ Practice soothing positions. Seated meditation, moderate neck stretches, and calm breathing help you relax.
- ❖ **Social Gatherings:** Subtly practice chair yoga during family gatherings or social events. There's no need to proclaim it; simply enjoy the rewards.
- ❖ **Practice Mindful Breathing Anytime:** The beauty of chair yoga is its versatility. When you're sitting, concentrate on your breath. Inhale deeply and expel fully. It's a miniature meditation.

Remember, consistency is more important than duration. ""Even dedicating just a few minutes each day can have a meaningful impact."."" as needed, and enjoy the process of incorporating chair yoga into your life.

Tips for Maintaining a Consistent Practice

To gain the benefits of chair yoga, you must practice it consistently. Whether you're a beginner, a senior, or an office worker, these practical recommendations can help you keep on track:

- ❖ **Establish a Routine:** Consistency is crucial. Make it a point to practice at the same time every day. Find a time that is convenient for you, whether it is in the morning, afternoon, or evening.
  - ➤ Make sure to warm up first, and then follow it with a cool down. Gentle stretches help prepare muscles and prevent soreness.
- ❖ **Focus on Breathing:** Pay attention to your breathing. Deep, consistent breathing promotes relaxation and concentration during chair yoga.
  - ➤ Use your breath as an anchor to be present and focused.
- ❖ **Pay Attention to Your Body:**
  - ➤ Start slowly and see how your body reacts. Do not force oneself into unpleasant stances.
  - ➤ Adjust as needed. If something feels stretched, make adjustments or skip it. Prioritize your own well-being.
- ❖ **Set Realistic Goals:**
  - ➤ Begin with shorter sessions if consistency is challenging. Even a few minutes per day count.
  - ➤ Gradually increase the duration of your practice until it becomes habitual.
- ❖ **Find a Supportive Space:**
  - ➤ Create a safe and comfortable location for chair yoga. Make sure your chair is solid and placed against a wall or on a yoga mat for traction.
  - ➤ Remove distractions to create a tranquil setting.
- ❖ **Incorporate Yoga into Daily Life:**
  - ➤ Integrate yoga into your lifestyle. Perform sun salutations in the morning or mild twists during work breaks.
  - ➤ Use waiting times or TV moments to do ankle circles or neck stretches.
- ❖ **Track Your Progress:**

➤ Use a journal or app to document your practice. Celebrate minor successes.

➤ Repetition improves consistency. Focus on one stance for a week before switching.

Reminisce that chair yoga adjusts to your requirements. These guidelines can help you keep a steady practice whether you're at home, in the workplace, or anyplace else.

Combining Chair Yoga with Other Wellness Practices

Combining chair yoga with other wellness activities can improve general health, induce relaxation, and increase quality of life.

 Let's look at how combining chair yoga with complementing activities can result in a more comprehensive approach:

❖ **Meditation and Mindfulness:**

➤ **Meditation:** After chair yoga, do meditation. Sit comfortably, close your eyes, and concentrate on your breathing or a relaxing mantra. Meditation improves mental clarity and lowers stress.

➤ **Mindfulness:** Be mindful throughout the day. Whether you're at your desk or waiting for an appointment, pay attention to your body, thoughts, and environment. Mindfulness enhances chair yoga by encouraging presence and stress reduction.

❖ **Breath work (Pranayama):**

➤ Practice pranayama methods during chair yoga. For example:

- ➤ **Deep Breathing:** Get comfortable in your chair, close your eyes, and take slow, deep breathes. Focus on the movement of your abdomen as it rises and falls.
- ➤ **Alternate Nostril Breathing:** With your thumb and ring finger, close one nostril at a time while inhaling and expelling through the other. This balances energy and relaxes the mind.
- ❖ **Hydration and Nutrition:** Stay hydrated. Drink water throughout chair yoga sessions to stay energized and improve joint health.
  - ➤ Eat healthy foods high in vitamins, minerals, and antioxidants. Proper diet complements physical exercise.
- ❖ **Self-Massage and Acupressure:**
  - ➤ Apply a tennis ball or massage roller on the backrest of your chair. Roll it along your spine to relieve tension.
  - ➤ Apply light pressure on the acupressure points on your hands, feet, and ears. These points represent numerous organs and systems in the body.
- ❖ **Visualization:** Combine chair yoga and visualization techniques. Imagine healing light or positive energy pouring through your body as you proceed through the positions. Visualization improves the mind-body link.
- ❖ **Aromatherapy:**
  - ➤ Apply a relaxing essential oil (such lavender or chamomile) to a tissue or cotton ball. Inhale the scent while practicing chair yoga. Aromatherapy encourages relaxation and emotional equilibrium.
- ❖ **Sound Healing:** Play relaxing music or nature sounds during your practice. Sound vibrations can boost the advantages of chair yoga and provide a relaxing environment. Put in mind that consistency is crucial. Gradually incorporate these routines into your everyday routine, tailoring them to your

own need. Chair yoga, when paired with other health practices, can result in overall well-being and a more vibrant existence.

Combining Chair Yoga and Other Wellness Practices

- ❖ **Synergy and Balance**
  - ➤ **Chair Yoga:** This mild type of yoga adapts conventional positions for persons who struggle to stand or go down on the floor.
  - ➤ It promotes physical, mental, and emotional health, making it suitable for people of all ages and abilities.
  - ➤ **Meditation:** Combining chair yoga and meditation promotes mindfulness, lowers stress, and increases relaxation.
  - ➤ **Massage:** Combining chair yoga and massage therapy can reduce tension, increase circulation, and improve the whole experience.
- ❖ **Physical benefits**
  Chair yoga increases flexibility, strength, and balance. Combining it with massage can improve muscular relaxation and joint mobility.
  - ➤ Meditation enhances chair yoga by encouraging relaxation and relieving muscle tension.
- ❖ **Mental and Emotional Wellbeing**
  - ➤ Chair yoga promotes feelings of community and belonging, both of which are beneficial to mental health.
  - ➤ Meditation improves mental clarity, lowers anxiety, and promotes self-awareness.

- ➤ Massage therapy produces endorphins, which promote emotional well-being.
- ❖ **Holistic Approach**
  - ➤ Combining these techniques leads to a comprehensive wellness regimen that includes physical, mental, and emotional elements.
  - ➤ Chair yoga, meditation, and massage work together to improve overall quality of life. To summarize, combining chair yoga with meditation and massage provides a holistic approach to wellbeing that benefits both the body and the mind. Whether you're a senior or looking for mild movement and relaxation, this integrative approach can improve your well-being.

Tracking Progress and Setting Goals

Let's look at the fundamentals of tracking progress and creating objectives in chair yoga. Whether you're a novice or an experienced practitioner, these techniques can help you improve your practice and general well-being.

Recording Progress in Chair Yoga

- ❖ **Journaling:** Keep a yoga journal and chronicle your everyday practice. Take note of the length, exact poses, and any alterations you make. Consider how you feel physically and emotionally after each session. Over time, this will assist you in identifying patterns, improvements, and growth opportunities.
- ❖ **Physical Markers:**
  - ➤ **Range of Motion:** Regularly evaluate joint flexibility and range of motion. Make note of any changes or limitations.

- ➢ **Strength:** Observe muscle strength gains, particularly in regions targeted by chair yoga postures.
- ➢ **Balance:** Monitor your ability to maintain balance while in positions. Gradual development is critical.

- ❖ **Mindfulness and Awareness:**
  - ➢ Focus on your breath, sensations, and thoughts during practice. Increased mindfulness improves self-awareness and progress monitoring.
  - ➢ Observe minor changes in energy, mood, and stress levels. These markers can suggest improvement that extends beyond bodily changes.

- ❖ **Goals for Chair Yoga**
- ❖ **Specificity:** Set clear and explicit goals. Avoid making ambiguous statements like ***"improve flexibility."*** Instead, make goals like "touch toes comfortably within six weeks."

- ❖ **SMART Goals:**
  - ➢ **Specific:** Define your desired outcome.
  - ➢ **Measurable:** Establish criteria to track progress (for example, hold a stance for 30 seconds).
  - ➢ **Achievable:** Make sure your goals are practical and reachable.
  - ➢ **Relevant:** Align goals with your entire health and lifestyle.
  - ➢ **Time-bound:** Establish a deadline (for example, complete a specific position by the end of the month).

- ❖ **Gradual Progression:**
  - ➢ Divide huge goals into smaller milestones. For example, if you want to improve your balance, begin with simple positions and work your way up.
  - ➢ Celebrate minor accomplishments along the way. Recognize progress, even if it appears modest.

- ❖ **Adaptability:** Be flexible in your goals. Life circumstances vary, and your practice should adjust accordingly.
  - ➢ Modify goals as necessary. If an accident happens, shift your focus to rehabilitation and healing.
- ❖ **Holistic Goals:**
  - ➢ Focus on mental and emotional well-being, in addition to physical health. Set goals for stress reduction, relaxation, and mindfulness.
  - ➢ Incorporate chair yoga into daily life, such as practicing mindful breathing during work breaks. Bear In Mind that your success in chair yoga is individualized and unique. Celebrate and honor your body's journey.

Success Stories and Testimonials

Let's look at amazing success stories and genuine testimonials from people who have tried chair yoga. Their experiences demonstrate the transformative potential of this peaceful practice, which promotes physical health, mental clarity, and emotional balance.

Success Stories and Testimonials for Chair Yoga

❖ **Grace's Transition to Mobility**

Grace, a vivacious 70-year-old, suffered from joint pain and reduced movement due to arthritis. Traditional yoga sessions seemed difficult, but she discovered chair yoga.

Below is her story:

I was hesitant at first about sitting in a chair and doing yoga. However, within weeks, I saw changes. My joints felt less tight, and I was able to reach objects on high shelves without suffering. The moderate stretches increased my flexibility, while the mindfulness aspect reduced my anxiousness. Now, I lead a weekly chair yoga session at our community center, encouraging people to discover their own grace."

❖ John's Stress Relief

John, a busy office worker, experienced stress, tension headaches, and bad posture.

❖ His testimonial highlights the impact of chair yoga:

My desk job had me crouched over a computer all day. Chair yoga became my lifeline. My stress headaches were eased by simple neck stretches, and deep breathing exercises helped to relax my thoughts. I also learned to sit with intention, which involved engaging my core and keeping a good posture. Now, my coworkers join me for lunch breaks, and we've established a 'Zen Zone' in the office.

❖ Maria's Emotional Healing

Maria, a retiree mourning the loss of her marriage, found peace in chair yoga.

She describes her heartfelt experience:

"After my spouse died, I felt adrift. Chair yoga became my retreat. The soothing motions helped me connect with my body and relieve emotional tension. Tears streamed down my cheeks at the 'heart-opening' stance, but it felt good. I gradually developed strength and resilience. Now, I volunteer at the senior center, educating others to this healing technique.

❖ Tom's Rehab Journey

Tom, who is recovering from knee surgery, discovered chair yoga as part of his recovery. His testimonial exemplifies determination and progress.

His story:

"After the surgery, I couldn't put weight on my knee. Chair yoga became my lifeline. The seated leg lifts and ankle circles helped to improve strength. I improved, I included standing postures with chair support. My surgeon credits chair yoga with my ability to walk pain-free today. It is not only physical, but also mental resilience.

❖ Sarah's Community Connection

Sarah, a young caregiver, discovered community and self-care through chair yoga. Her tale resonates with many people.

Her story:

"Being a caretaker exhausted me emotionally. Chair yoga courses at a nearby community center were my retreat. The friendship, laughing, and shared experiences boosted my spirits. I learnt to breathe deeply even in the midst of pandemonium. Now, I organize **'Caregivers'** *Wellness Circles,' in which we practice chair yoga together. It's our lifeline, a reminder that we are not alone.* These success stories and testimonials demonstrate the worldwide attraction of chair yoga. Whether you're a senior seeking gentle movement, an office worker dealing with stress, or on a healing journey, chair yoga provides a seat of transformation.

CONCLUSION

Thank you for joining us on this journey through the world of chair yoga for seniors over 60. As you close this book, I invite you to reflect on the wisdom and gentle movements you've discovered within these pages.

Always remember, wellness is not a sprint; it's a marathon. Just as a tree grows slowly, day by day, so too does our well-being. Consistency in practicing chair yoga will yield remarkable results over time. Whether you're easing joint pain, improving flexibility, or simply finding moments of peace, trust that each session contributes to your overall health.

Good things take time. As you settle into your practice, embrace patience. Allow yourself to progress at your own pace. Some days, you might feel like a sprightly gazelle; other days, a graceful tortoise. Both are valid. Celebrate every small victory—the extra inch of stretch, the deeper breath, the quieting of the mind.

Take a moment to appreciate your body. It has carried you through decades of life, and now, with each mindful movement, it continues to serve you. Express gratitude for its resilience, and honor it by showing up on the mat regularly.

If this book has touched your heart, consider leaving your honest review. Your words can inspire others to explore the benefits of chair yoga. By sharing your experience, you contribute to a ripple effect of well-being that extends far beyond these pages.

Together, We Thrive As the author, I am deeply grateful for your trust and engagement. Your commitment to self-care fuels my passion to create more resources like this. Let's continue this journey together, supporting one another as we age gracefully and mindfully.

With heartfelt appreciation,

Ruth Sinclair-